PUBLIC HEALTH IN THE 21ST CENTURY

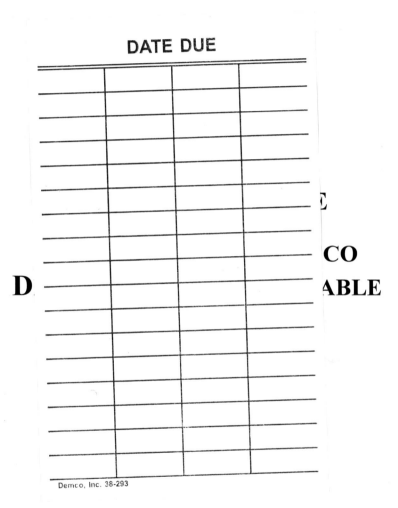

DATE DUE

PUBLIC HEALTH IN THE 21ST CENTURY

Additional books in this series can be found on Nova's website at:

https://www.novapublishers.com/catalog/index.php?cPath=23_29&seriesp=
Public+Health+in+the+21st+Century

Additional E-books in this series can be found on Nova's website at:

https://www.novapublishers.com/catalog/index.php?cPath=23_29&seriespe=
Public+Health+in+the+21st+Century

BREAKING DOWN BARRIERS TO CARE

TREATMENT OF TOBACCO DEPENDENCE IN VULNERABLE POPULATIONS

JOHN E. SNYDER

AND

MEGAN J. ENGELEN

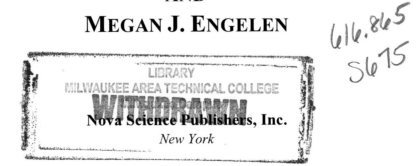

Nova Science Publishers, Inc.

New York

For permission to use material from this book please contact us:
Telephone 631-231-7269; Fax 631-231-8175
Web Site: http://www.novapublishers.com

NOTICE TO THE READER

LIBRARY OF CONGRESS CATALOGING-IN-PUBLICATION DATA
Engelen, Megan J.
Treating tobacco dependence in vulnerable populations / authors, Megan J. Engelen and John E. Snyder.
p. ; cm.
Includes bibliographical references and index.
ISBN 978-1-60876-976-6 (softcover)
1. Smoking. 2. Nicotine addiction--Treatment. I. Snyder, John E. II. Title.
[DNLM: 1. Tobacco Use Disorder--therapy--United States. 2. Tobacco Use Cessation--methods--United States. 3. Vulnerable Populations--United States. WM 290 E57t 2009]
HV5740.E54 2009
616.86'506--dc22
2009049859

Published by Nova Science Publishers, Inc. ✛ *New York*

CONTENTS

PREFACE

Although entirely preventable, smoking is one of the most common causes of morbidity and mortality in the United States. As a result it creates a significant financial burden on the health care system. In the text, the authors first present an evidence-based approach for providers that helps identify the most at-risk patients. They then offer specific clinical strategies for approaching tobacco cessation which are proven to be the most effective in overcoming the existing cultural or systematic barriers. Lastly, the authors propose a number of health policy recommendations which can assist with breaking down barriers to care for each cultural group and result in more effective cessation programs on the population level.

Although this text is clearly about the treatment of tobacco dependence, the authors hope that the subtext about providing the highest-possible quality of culturally-competent care, with due consideration to public health contexts, carries through loudly and clearly. Through a better understanding of cultural perspectives, and an open-eyed awareness of existing health care barriers, an individual's health care needs can ultimately be far better served by their provider.

FOREWORD:
TOBACCO CONTROL IN A "FLAT WORLD" – GLOBALIZATION AND NEW PUBLIC HEALTH PERSPECTIVES

In his insightful 2005 book *The World is Flat: A Brief History of the Twenty-First Century*, Thomas Friedman described how the digital age, transportation, political change, and economic influences have hastened "globalism" – an intermingling and unification of people from all countries and walks of life [1]. One can simply pick up a phone and join a conference call between the United States, China, and South Africa. In a mere instant, information can be digitally transmitted from one part of the world to another. And within hours, a person can travel from one end of the globe to another. These technologies are advancing at a lightning pace, and their impact on the world is just in the beginning stages. As people from diverse backgrounds and cultures become interconnected, the peace, health, and well-being of people from different nations are also joined [2]. From the public health perspective, the implications can be enormous. If someone with an infectious disease, like Severe Acute Respiratory Syndrome (SARS), gets on a plane from Beijing to New York, an illness can quickly transform from outbreak to epidemic and pandemic proportions [3]. The World Health Organization has had, as a result, to form a Global Outbreak Alert and Response Network to adjust to such problems [4]. The health problems of previously distant parts of the world are no longer so isolated and ignorable has they have been considered to be in the past [2].

Some critics of *The World is Flat* claim that the world is, in the current economic climate, not flat but "tilted" in the favor of large corporations who exploit nations where labor costs are low and greater profits can be acquired [5].

Other tactics of such corporations can have major impacts on public health. Take "Big Tobacco" as an example: in countries where health policy is not as progressive or established as it is in Western nations, transnational tobacco companies have found a way to reap huge profits and offset the declines in tobacco product consumption observed in more developed areas [6]. Enormous marketing campaigns over the last two decades have promoted tobacco use in these countries, and the health implications of this advertising are enormous. It is anticipated that by the year 2030, there will be 7 million deaths annually in developing countries that are attributable to tobacco use [7]. Up to 18.3% of pregnant women in Latin American countries are active smokers, and second-hand smoke exposure rates are high as well, affecting both maternal and child health [8]. The effectiveness of cessation aids in developing nations is not known, and the cost of such aids in these countries may be prohibitive [9].

Whether you believe that the world is "flat" or if it's "tilted," both theories come to the same conclusion about the health implications of tobacco dependence in an increasingly "globalized" world. Tobacco companies are finding alternative means for profit – and countless lives are being lost as a result. Few public health problems are rooted in such a profit-hungry business model, and "Big Tobacco" must be stopped. We must no longer ignore the health of developing nations. We are connected to and dependent on their welfare as much as they are on ours. International efforts are clearly going to be necessary to reverse the pandemic-like spread of tobacco-related disease across other nations. Policy initiatives to prevent tobacco-related disease must occur globally, locally, and everywhere in between.

REFERENCES

[1]   Friedman T. *The world is flat*. New York: Farrar, Straus and Giroux; 2005.

[2]   Spencer DC. The neurology world is flat. *Neurology*. 2007 Oct 23;69(17):E16-7. Comment on: *Neurology*. 2007 Oct 23. 69(17):1715-8.

[3]   Severe Acute Respiratory Syndrome (SARS). Retrieved June 13, 2009 from: http://www.who.int/csr/sars/en/index.html.

[4]   Global Outbreak Alert and Response Network. Retrieved June 13, 2009 from: http://www.who.int/csr/outbreaknetwork/en/.

[5]   Aronica R, Ramdoo M. *The World Is Flat?: A Critical Analysis of New York Times Bestseller by Thomas Friedman*. Meghan-Kiffer Press;2006.

[6]   Stebbins KR. Going like Gangbusters: Transnational Tobacco Companies "Making a Killing" in South America. *Medical Anthropology Quarterly*, New Series. June 2001. 15(2): 147-170.

[7]   Dobson R. Annual tobacco deaths in poor countries to reach 7 million by 2030. *BMJ*. July 10, 2004. 329: 71.

[8]   Bloch M, Althabe F, Onyamboko M, Kaseba-Sata C, Castilla EE, Freire S, Garces AL, Parida S, Goudar SS, Kadir MM, Goco N, Thornberry J, Daniels M, Bartz J, Hartwell T, Moss N, Goldenberg R. Tobacco Use and Secondhand Smoke Exposure During Pregnancy: An Investigative Survey of Women in 9 Developing Nations. *American Journal of Public Health*. October 2008. 98:1833-1840.

[9]   Abdullah ASM, Husten CG. Promotion of smoking cessation in developing countries: a framework for urgent public health interventions. *Thorax*. 2004. 59:623-630.

PART I.
CULTURAL BARRIERS
TO TREATING TOBACCO DEPENDENCE

CULTURAL BARRIERS TO TREATING TOBACCO DEPENDENCE – INTRODUCTION

Although entirely preventable, smoking is one of the most common causes of morbidity and mortality in the United States. As a result it creates a significant financial burden on the health care system. This creates an obligation and urgency on the part of health care providers, public health officials, and government leaders to address the causes of smoking and identify the populations most susceptible, common barriers to quitting smoking, and strategies for improving success rates of cessation. Tobacco policy must address all of these concerns. To most effectively accomplish these tasks we must better understand influences that encourage smoking and barriers to successful cessation in at-risk patient populations. This requires a multifaceted, individualized, and culturally-sensitive approach.

Patients in certain at-risk cultural groups are uniquely vulnerable to tobacco dependence for many reasons. Factors such as directed and aggressive tobacco industry marketing techniques, barriers to accessing health care providers who provide treatment for tobacco dependence, inequitable access to pharmacological treatment options, and a limited availability of culture-specific support resources play significant roles. In the first part of this book, we identify six distinctive patient subpopulations, each with unique cultural characteristics to consider during the effective treatment of tobacco dependence. These include patient groups based on a patient's gender, age, race and ethnicity, native language, and sexual orientation. We first present an evidence-based approach for providers that helps identify the most at-risk patients. We then offer specific clinical strategies for approaching tobacco cessation which are proven to be the most effective in overcoming the existing cultural barriers. Lastly, we propose a number of health policy recommendations which can assist with breaking down barriers to care for each cultural group and result in more effective cessation programs on the population level.

Chapter 1

TOBACCO DEPENDENCE TREATMENT AND CULTURE

In 2006 the Centers for Disease Control estimated that about 21% of the United States population currently smoked tobacco [1]. The health impacts of tobacco dependence are vast and create a burden on society in caring for the people who develop chronic and life-threatening diseases as a consequence of smoking. Although overall 70% of smokers express a desire to quit, only about 2.5 million out of the 30 million total smokers who each year attempt to quit are successful [2]. Since the success rate of quitting smoking is so low, and the morbidity and mortality associated with tobacco dependence is so high, it has become a national health priority to address prevention, cessation, and the barriers that prevent people from quitting smoking. The health benefits that can be achieved from tobacco cessation are very cost-effective. Studies suggest that the estimated cost-per-life-year saved ranges from $2,300-4,200 [3]. In comparison, screening and treatment for hypertension costs $14,000-30,000 per quality-adjusted life year.

Treatment of tobacco dependence in clinical practice is best served by using the "five A's." They are: *Ask* about smoking, *Advise* smokers to quit, *Assess* readiness to quit, *Assist* patients to quit, and *Arrange* follow-up [4] (*see Figure 1.1*). The provider interventions that tend to lead to increased success rates include when the physician or other health care provider always asks about the patient's desire to quit smoking *and* advises them to quit, when the provider refers the patient to tobacco cessation resources such as a telephone quit line or behavioral counseling, and when the provider offers the patient nicotine replacement or other pharmacotherapy [4]. Studies suggest that 28% of patients will quit when they have access to both professional counseling and pharmaceutical aides [5] – over three times the current national quit rate [2].

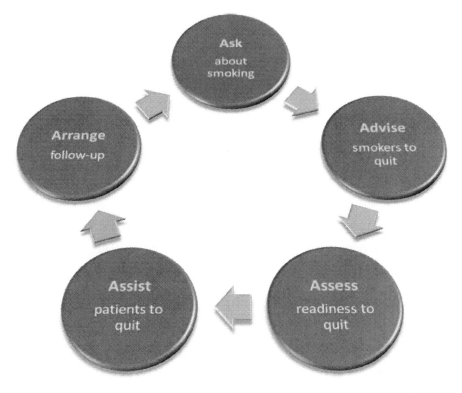

Figure 1.1. The "five A's:" a proven approach to treatment of tobacco dependence in clinical practice.

As smoking cessation often involves repeated quit attempts interjected with periods of relapse, it is important to note that continued intensive support programs, with the assistance of pharmacotherapeutic agents, may lead to greater periods of abstinence [5]. Generally, with the right support, most smokers are willing to continue trying to quit smoking with this high-intensity level of disease management.

However, not all patients will respond similarly to different tobacco cessation strategies. Therein lies the challenge for providers, as assisting individuals with tobacco dependence requires a customized approach to prevention, education, and assistance with cessation. Patient cultural factors additionally seem to play an important role in successful tobacco cessation. Culture is a broad term, defined as "the sum of attitudes, customs, and beliefs that distinguishes one group of people from another ... [sic] ... transmitted through language, material objects, ritual, institutions, and art, from one generation to the next [6]. Cultural groups include those united by similarities such as those of gender, age, race, ethnicity, sexual orientation, religion, geography, native language, and socioeconomic status – among others, such as shared life experiences. Cultural factors play an important and increasingly recognized role in an individual's belief system, and understanding a patient's cultural background may help aide in individualizing their medical needs and optimizing their care.

The effect of patient cultural background appears to be particularly important when it comes to the treatment of tobacco dependence. Both differences in the prevalence of tobacco use and in the success rates of different cessation techniques seem to exist among different culturally-based subpopulations of patients. In addition, there is also a discrepancy seen in the frequency of tobacco cessation counseling done by physicians to patients in different sociocultural subpopulations. For example, women, ethnic minorities, persons with Medicaid, and patients who are uninsured are all less likely to receive appropriate tobacco counseling and cessation services by physicians [7]. Due to the health consequences of smoking, those in the medical profession and in the public health field need to work harder to augment the number of people who try and successfully quit smoking. But in order to accomplish this task, we must better understand the factors associated with smoking in specific target patient populations as well as the barriers of these patients to successfully quit smoking.

REFERENCES

[1]   U.S. Centers for Disease Control and Prevention (CDC), "Cigarette Smoking in Adults – -- United States 2006." *Morbidity and Mortality Weekly Report (MMWR).* November 9, 2007. 56(44):1157-1161. Acquired on June 4, 2009 at: http://www.cdc.gov/mmwr/preview/mmwrhtml/mm5644a2. htm.

[2]   Gollust S, Schroeder S, Warner K. Helping Smokers Quit: Understanding the Barriers to Utilization of Smoking Cessation Services. *The Milbank Quarterly*, 2008. 86(4):601-627.

[3]   Warner KE, Mendez D, Smith DG. The Financial Implications of Coverage of Smoking Cessation Treatment by Managed Care Organizations. 2004. Inquiry 41 (1): 57-69.

[4] Fiore MC, Bailey WC, Cohen SF. 2000. Treating Tobacco Use and Dependence: A Clinical Practice Guideline. Rockville, MD. U.S. Department of Health and Human Services.

[5] Ellerbeck EF, Mahnken JD, Cupertino P, Sanderson Cox L, Greiner KA, Mussulman LM, Nazir N, Shireman TI, Resnicow K, Ahluwalia JS. Effect of Varying Levels of Disease Management on Smoking Cessation: A Randomized Trial. *Annals of Internal Medicine.* 2009. 150(7):437-446.

[6] culture. (n.d.). *The American Heritage® New Dictionary of Cultural Literacy, Third Edition.* Retrieved May 17, 2009, from Dictionary.com website: http://dictionary1.classic.reference.com/browse/culture

[7] Report of the Surgeon General on Tobacco Use Among US Racial/Ethnic Minority Groups. Washington DC : US Department of Health and Human Services 1998.

Chapter 2

TOBACCO DEPENDENCE TREATMENT AND FEMALE GENDER

TOBACCO USE PATTERNS AND PUBLIC HEALTH IMPACT

Males have always been more prevalent smokers than females. In the most recent survey by the Centers for Disease Control, the smoking rate for men is 22.3% and for women is 17.4% [1]. Even though males have a higher prevalence of smoking, these rates have decreased by 50% since the 1960's, whereas the prevalence of smoking in females has only decreased by 38% in that same period [2]. The highest prevalence of female smokers is amongst American Indian or Alaska Native women (34.5%), then white women (23.5%), then black women (21.9%). The lowest prevalence is among Hispanic (13.8%) and Asian women (11.2%) [3] (*see Figure 2.1*). Additionally, women who have achieved a lower education level (9-11 years of school) have a prevalence rate of 30.9%, and those with 16 or more years of school have a 10.6% prevalence rate of smoking [3].

An important reason for cessation in both men and women is that heart disease is the primary cause of death in the United States and smoking contributes to the morbidity and mortality of heart disease. There are also specific health consequences of smoking that tend to disproportionately affect women (*see Table 2.1*). Young female smokers tend to have more significant early deleterious changes in their lung function, noted during pulmonary function testing, than their male counterparts [4]. In women who are actively smoking, the annual risk of death is double that of their non-smoking peers, and they have an average of a 14 year shorter lifespan [3].

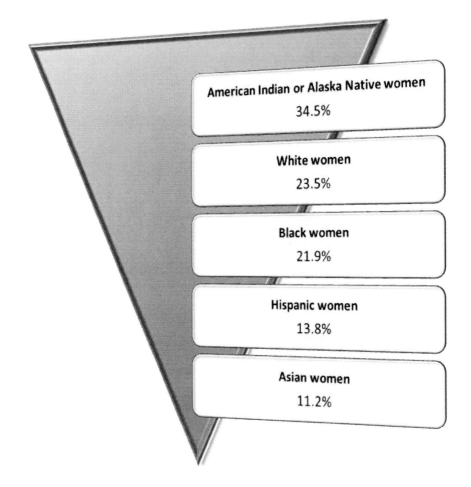

Figure 2.1. The prevalence of smoking among women, with regard to their racial and ethnic background.

Lung cancer rates have increased 600% in women over the last 50 years, surpassing breast cancer as the most common cause of cancer death in women [3]. The lung cancer rate in black females is 42.6 cases per 100,000 population and in white females is 45 cases per 100,000 population [3]. Women who smoke are also at higher risk for cervical and vulvar cancer, stroke, heart disease, peripheral vascular disease, colon cancer, pancreatic cancer, dysmenorrhea, menstrual irregularities, infertility, ectopic pregnancy, decreased bone mineral density, and increased risk of hip fracture, among other problems [5].

Table 2.1. Health consequences of smoking that tend to disproportionately or solely affect women

Health consequences that disproportionately or solely affect women:
early deleterious changes in lung function
cervical and vulvar cancer
stroke
heart disease
peripheral vascular disease
colon cancer
pancreatic cancer
dysmenorrheal
menstrual irregularities
decreased bone mineral density
increased risk of hip fracture

Health consequences related to pregnancy and to the unborn child:
infertility
ectopic pregnancy
low birth weight
premature rupture of membranes/preterm delivery
abruptio placentae
placenta previa

Tobacco dependence treatment is critical in women not only for the overall adverse health effects for themselves, but also for the consequences in pregnancy and to the unborn child. There have been countless studies on the negative effects of smoking on the fetus, including low birth weight, premature rupture of membranes/preterm delivery, abruptio placentae, and placenta previa [6].

POPULATION-SPECIFIC BARRIERS TO TREATMENT OF TOBACCO DEPENDENCE

Women tend to be influenced by factors that diminish smoking avoidance, limit successful cessation, and that are unique from men. Studies suggest that women are often influenced by the advertising media's depiction of desirable, attractive, and independent women in cigarette ads that portray themes of social desirability and independence, even though the consequences of smoking are much the opposite [3]. Tobacco advertising also targets women by sponsorship of women's fashion, artistic, athletic, and political events [3]. Data also suggest that women are more likely to continue smoking due to the desire to be thin and the thought that quitting smoking will cause them to gain weight [7], [8]. Women also generally have a tendency to need more social support in quitting tobacco [5]. Patient gender can often additionally play a role in access to general medical care. Numerous studies show that a woman's health and nutrition are often devalued and that female patients do not always receive the same medical treatments as male counterparts [see, for example, 6].

CLINICAL SOLUTIONS

Clinical recommendations for treating women smokers include involving them in counseling and support groups, referring them for cognitive behavioral therapy, offering them pharmacological interventions such as bupropion and varenicline, and encouraging them to partake in adjunctive exercise programs. Significant gender-based differences in long-term cessation rates when using the nicotine patch have been seen. In one clinical study, women had worse outcomes than men when treated with the nicotine patch, whether or not formal counseling was also provided [9]. Multiple other clinical trials have compared the efficacy of nicotine replacement therapy in the quit rates of women versus men. Some of these studies have found that these treatments are less successful in maintaining long-term abstinence in women compared with men [2]. Gender-based differences seen in the efficacy of nicotine replacement treatment can be partly explained by the fact that women may tend to experience more severe nicotine withdrawal symptoms and also greater adverse effects of nicotine replacement therapy than men [2]. Women have a tendency to have lower compliance rates with this treatment, as well as a higher attachment to the behaviors associated with smoking beyond simply the addiction to nicotine [2].

Bupropion has been studied in women and most placebo-controlled trials show no gender differences in tobacco cessation with this medication. A prospective trial showed that, in pregnancy, giving bupropion was associated with a 45% quit rate as compared with a 14% quit rate in controls [10]. Gender differences in varenicline therapy have been evaluated in at least one clinical trial, which showed that abstinence rates for men and women at 9-12 weeks were equivocal [11].

In women, there is a high association of weight gain with smoking cessation. This precludes many women from quitting, and may also decrease the long term compliance if there is subsequent weight gain [12]. Studies have found that not only is there a higher tobacco cessation rate but also that actual weight loss is associated with multifaceted smoking cessation programs that include a combination of exercise, counseling, and nicotine replacement therapy [12].

When choosing pharmacotherapeutic agents for female smokers of child-bearing age, it is important to consider the drugs' safety profiles during pregnancy and breast-feeding. In general, women who are pregnant or breast-feeding should attempt smoking cessation without the use of medications. Bupropion [13] and varenicline [14] have not been adequately studied in pregnant or lactating women. They are both currently classified in pregnancy class 'C' and should be used during pregnancy only if the potential benefit justifies the potential risk to the fetus. Bupropion is secreted in human milk, and it is not known if the same occurs for varenicline; generally neither should be taken while breast feeding. Nicotine replacement aides are believed to be safer than smoking in pregnancy, however the risks of using such products during pregnancy or breast-feeding are not completely understood [15]. The use of any pharmacotherapeutic agent for tobacco cessation during pregnancy or lactation should be done with extreme caution and only with the explicit direction of a patient's provider.

HEALTH POLICY RECOMMENDATIONS

There are many opportunities to affect health policy for tobacco dependence in women. Programs to counteract female-targeted advertising, and particularly geared toward young women, may aid in greater smoking prevention. Initiatives such as the youth-oriented 'TheTruth.com' campaign tend to focus on racial diversity, but could be easily adapted to be more gender-based. Educating primary care providers to remember to counsel women on smoking cessation and on what techniques are most effective for women is essential.

Policy also should be targeted at tobacco cessation during pregnancy and on maintaining that cessation thereafter. Currently one-third of women who quit tobacco during pregnancy go back to using tobacco after they have delivered [6]. Hospitalization for labor and delivery is an important opportunity to impact the smoking rates of women, because they are unlikely to be able to smoke while in the hospital, and they can be encouraged to maintain tobacco cessation for the health and wellbeing of their newborn child. Implementing a multi-faceted post-partum support plan for new mothers who quit smoking, including close primary care follow-up, would likely be the key to the success of such an initiative. This is particularly true given the stress, exhaustion, "maternity blues," and even post-partum depression that can follow childbirth. Additionally, increasing the number of and access to prenatal and postnatal support groups could improve adherence to cessation. Studies suggest that women may be more influenced by emotional ties than men, and hence may need stronger social support systems during smoking cessation [11].

KEY POINTS

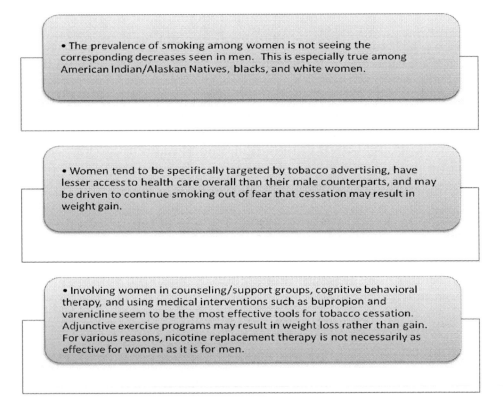

- The prevalence of smoking among women is not seeing the corresponding decreases seen in men. This is especially true among American Indian/Alaskan Natives, blacks, and white women.

- Women tend to be specifically targeted by tobacco advertising, have lesser access to health care overall than their male counterparts, and may be driven to continue smoking out of fear that cessation may result in weight gain.

- Involving women in counseling/support groups, cognitive behavioral therapy, and using medical interventions such as bupropion and varenicline seem to be the most effective tools for tobacco cessation. Adjunctive exercise programs may result in weight loss rather than gain. For various reasons, nicotine replacement therapy is not necessarily as effective for women as it is for men.

- Counteracting gender-based tobacco advertising, increasing primary care-based interventions, and assisting female smokers in the peri-partum period are key to successful health policy initiatives for women.

REFERENCES

[1]   U.S. Centers for Disease Control and Prevention (CDC), "Cigarette Smoking Among Adults- United States 2007." *Morbidity and Mortality Weekly Report (MMWR)*. Nov 14, 2008. 57(45): 1221-1226. Acquired on June 4, 2009 at *http://www.cdc.gov/mmwr/preview/mmwrhtml/ mm5745a2.htm.*

[2]   Schnoll RA, Patterson F, Lerman C. Treating Tobacco Dependence in Women. *Journal of Women's Health.* Nov. 8, 2007. 16(8): 1211-1217.

[3]   Office of the Surgeon General. Women and smoking: A Report of the Surgeon General. Retrieved June 4, 2009 from: http://www.surgeongeneral. gov/library/womenandtobacco/.

[4]   Woolf A. Smoking and Nicotine Addiction: A Pediatric Epidemic with Sequelae in Adulthood. *Current Opinion in Pediatrics.* 1997. 9:470-477.

[5]   U.S. Centers for Disease Control and Prevention (CDC), " Women and smoking: A Report of the Surgeon General. Chapter 5: Efforts to reduce tobacco use among women." *Morbidity and Mortality Weekly Report (MMWR).* August 30, 2002. 51(RR12):1-30. Acquired on June 4, 2009 at: http://www.cdc.gov/mmwr/preview/mmwrhtml/rr5112a4.htm.

[6]   World Health Organization. Gender or women's health: why should WHO work on this? WHO role as an advocate for gender equality and women's health. Retrieved June 4, 2009 from: http://www.who.int/gender/about/ gender_or_womens_health/en/index.html.

[7]   Levine MD, Perkins KA, Marcus MD. The Characteristics of Women Smokers Concerned about Postcessation Weight Gain. *Addicitive Behaviors.* 2001. 26(5):749-756.

[8]   Clark MM, Hurt RD, Croghan IT, Patten CA, Novotny P, Sloan JA, Dakhil SR et al. The Prevalence of Weight Concerns in a Smoking Abstinence Clinical Trial. *Addictive Behaviors.* 2006. 31(7):1144-1152.

[9]   Perkins KA, Scott J. Sex differences in long-term smoking cessation rates due to nicotine patch. *Nicotine and Tobacco Research.* 2008 Jul. 10(7):1245-50.

[10] Chan B, Einarson A, Koren G. Effectiveness of bupropion for smoking cessation during pregnancy. *Journal of Addictive Diseases.* 2005. 20:19.

[11] Gonzales D, Rennard SI, Nides M, Oncken C, Azoulay S, Billing CB, Watsky EJ, Gong J, Williams KE, Reeves KR. Varenicline, an $\alpha4\beta2$ Nicotinic Acetylcholine Receptor Partial Agonist, vs Sustained-Release Bupropion and Placebo for Smoking Cessation: A Randomized Controlled Trial. 2006. *JAMA.* 296: 47-55.

[12] Chaney SE, Sheriff S. Weight Gain Among Women During Smoking Cessation: Testing the Effects of a Multifaceted Program. *AAOHN Journal*. March 2008. 56(3).

[13] Prescribing Information: CHANTIX® (varenicline) Tablets. Dosage and Administration. Retrieved May 17, 2009 from https://www.pfizerpro. com/sites/pfp/pages/product_info/Chantix_pi_dosage_and_adminiadminist. aspx and http://www.pfizer.com/files/products/uspi_chantix.pdf.

[14] Bupropion hydrochloride drug information. Retrieved May 17, 2009 from http://www.fda.gov/cder/drug/infopage/bupropion/default.htm.

[15] Nicorette Stop Smoking Gum. Frequently asked questions. Retrieved May 24, 2009 from http://www.nicorette.com/Faqs.aspx#21 and http://www. nicorette.com/Nicorette_Know.aspx.

Chapter 3

TOBACCO DEPENDENCE TREATMENT IN ADOLESCENTS AND YOUNG ADULTS

TOBACCO USE PATTERNS AND PUBLIC HEALTH IMPACT

Adolescent and young adult smoking is quite prevalent, estimated at a rate of about 21.9% in 2003, and most smokers start using tobacco before they are 18 years old [1], [2]. Fortunately, these rates represent an overall decline from the 36.4% prevalence rate seen in 1997 [2]. Tobacco use rates are highest among white youths (30.9%) when compared to African American (12.6%) and Hispanic youth (25.3%). The Surgeon General's Report on youth and smoking from 1994 revealed that an increased risk of smoking in adolescents and young adults was associated with family structure. Youth who lived alone were the most likely to smoke, followed by those who lived in a single parent home in which the mother was absent, and then by youth who were home alone while their parents worked [1]. The report also noted an inverse relationship between smoking and population density, with the highest smoking rates seen in rural areas [1]. The lowest smoking rates were seen in youth with plans for attending college after high school graduation and in those with strong religious beliefs [1]. Smoking initiation also seems to be associated with inadequate parental monitoring, homes in which the parents are smoking, and having peers and friends who smoke [3]. Most of the factors that tend to contribute to youth smoking are universal throughout different socioeconomic levels and demographic groups. The key underlying theme is that youth who have role models (such as parents and peer influences) that smoke may find it harder to understand the reasons to never start smoking, or to appreciate the long-term health consequences of smoking.

The immediate health impacts of youth tobacco use are increased rates of chronic cough, acute bronchitis, and chest illness [3]. Young smokers, and in particular young females, can often already demonstrate detrimental changes in lung function as seen by pulmonary function testing [3]. In addition to causing a shortened life expectancy, many of the specific negative health effects from smoking have a dose-response relationship. Cancer of the nasopharynx, larynx, lung, esophagus, stomach, pancreas, bladder, and cervix all tend to have such an association, and are related to long-term tobacco use [3]. Hence, youth and adolescents have the greatest potential for long-term harms from the initiation of smoking.

POPULATION-SPECIFIC BARRIERS TO TREATMENT OF TOBACCO DEPENDENCE

Although a visit to the pediatrician's office provides an occasion to counsel on smoking prevention and cessation, many pediatricians do not routinely address tobacco use with their patients [4]. If they do, they are more likely to counsel their patients on prevention rather than discuss cessation. Many adolescents may not be honest with their providers about their use of tobacco, and an opportunity for tobacco dependence treatment is lost.

Despite this, studies have found that 75% of high school students who smoke have tried to quit smoking, and that most students are interested in cessation [5]. However, certain unique barriers to successful cessation exist in the adolescent and young adult population. For one, youth may be less likely to identify themselves as a "smoker" because they may only smoke when they are with friends or if they feel the need to fit in with a crowd [6]. When polled, most adolescents who currently smoke do not believe they will continue to do so long-term [4]. However, even "social" tobacco use may lead to more regular smoking and eventual addiction. Between 33 and 50% of adolescents who experiment with tobacco become regular smokers [1]. Studies suggest that 75% of current youth smokers are still smoking when re-polled five years later [4]. Despite an intention to not smoke long-term, or even a belief that "social" smoking is not a habit, many youth still seem to become dependent on tobacco in this way.

Youth and young adults seem to be one of the most vulnerable populations to the influences of peer pressure, directed advertising, and the presence of tobacco in entertainment and other media [6], [7], [8]. Studies have demonstrated that cartoon characters used in tobacco advertising, such as "Joe Camel," are not only easily recognizable by minors but also are strongly associated with the initiation of tobacco use [8], [9]. In movies, for another example, the smoking message is more hidden and therefore doesn't get the same criticism as direct advertising to youth from tobacco companies [10]. A study of the top-grossing twenty-five films in the U.S., in each year over a ten year period from 1988 to 1997, found tobacco use in 85% of the films and the presence of brand name products in 28% [11]. Brand products were present even in 20% of the films that were specifically rated for children. Despite 1998 settlement agreements prohibiting tobacco manufacturers from paid advertising of brand tobacco products in movies, television, video games, or similar media [12], these products still find their way into such media outlets. In the top five grossing U.S. films of 2000, there were an average of 10.9 instances of smoking per hour, compared to 7.3 instances in the top films of 1960 [13], [14]. In one study, a dose-response relationship was measured between exposure to movie smoking and initiation of smoking in youth [10]. Households with children tend to watch an average of three movies per week [10]. Movie stars may be inspirational role models for children and adolescents, and stars that smoke on-screen may be sending the message to youth that smoking is socially desirable. Tobacco companies have also targeted general-audience public entertainment venues such as sporting events, spending $30.6 million on these events in 2005 [15]. Star athletes likely have similar social influences on youth as movie actors.

Evidence is mounting that directed tobacco industry marketing also strengthens cigarette addiction in young adults, in a time period where experimentation may occur and lead to more regular usage [16]. A Cochrane Systematic Review examining nine longitudinal studies and including over 12,000 youth concluded that nonsmoking adolescents with greater exposure to and receptiveness toward this sort of marketing are more likely to eventually become smokers [17]. Promotions often target youth and young adults via the military, colleges, the workplace, and bars [16]. Cigarette brands that are more popular in young smokers are more heavily advertised in magazines with high readership in this age group [18]. College students are a particularly frequent target of tobacco industry promotions. In one study of 119 colleges and universities [19], 99.2% of students reported the presence of tobacco-sponsored social events at bars, nightclubs, or on campus where free cigarettes were distributed. Attendance rates at these events were approximately 8.5%, and attendance was associated with higher prevalence rates of smoking.

CLINICAL SOLUTIONS

In pediatrics and adolescent medicine, there is a great opportunity to intervene in smoking prevention and cessation. One reason is that, in most states, children under 18 are covered by state health insurance plans and hence have access to affordable medical care even if they are in a low socioeconomic class. Also, between 63-85% of adolescents are seen for preventive care each year [4]. Since access to affordable care is a lesser problem in this patient population, there is a greater opportunity to screen for tobacco use and to intervene early on smoking cessation. Pediatricians usually have a long-term relationship with their patients and may have a greater influence on certain risk behaviors than even the patient's parents.

Evidence suggests that the best clinical solutions for tobacco cessation in adolescents and young adults include the use of nicotine replacement therapy (such as the nicotine patch), counseling, and cognitive-behavioral therapy. The rates of tobacco cessation by adolescents with the patch are similar to that of the adult population [6]. However, it is important to note that the sale of nicotine and nicotine-containing products such as gum is prohibited in persons under 18 years of age in the United States [20]. In addition to nicotine replacement therapy, there are other strategies to tobacco cessation in adolescents. Counseling from health care providers and peers can improve quit rates [4]. It has also been shown that cognitive behavioral therapy can improve cessation in adolescents and young adults [21]. Evidence also overall supports the clinical benefit of computer- and internet-based smoking cessation programs [22], which may appeal to youth who have grown up with these technologies and may be more savvy with them.

A randomized controlled trial looked at practice-based smoking prevention and cessation techniques for adolescents using the "5A approach" and included referring patients to peer counselors in order to develop a personalized approach for cessation or sustained abstinence [4]. Counseling was first done in-person, and then with follow-up phone conversations four times over the next 5 months. For the non-smokers in the trial, 95.5% in the usual care group continued to be abstinent at 12 months, compared with 96.8% in the intervention group. Quit rates for smokers were 24.6% at six months' time in the usual care cohort, and 36.4% in the intervention group. However, at 12 months the sustained quit rates were 27.7% and 25.3%, respectively. One might infer from this study that provider-initiated cessation, supplemented with counseling, can improve young adults' cessation rates, but only in the first few months after intervention. There needs to be continued and frequent re-evaluation and abstinence counseling to improve the long term cessation rates in this population.

Pharmacological treatment of tobacco dependence in persons less than 18 years of age, and particularly with bupropion [23] and varenicline [24], is currently limited since the safety and efficacy of these agents have not been well-studied in younger patients. These agents are not currently approved by the FDA for tobacco dependence treatment in this population. Although bupropion has been studied in adolescents, and its side effect profile was felt to be tolerable, it has not been consistently demonstrated to increase smoking cessation in this population [25], [26]. Anti-depressants, such as bupropion, also carry a "black box" warning that they may increase suicidal thoughts and actions in about 1 out of 50 people who are 18 years old or younger [23].

HEALTH POLICY RECOMMENDATIONS

The health impact of tobacco addiction at an early age is a significant public health crisis. It is critically important to understand what influences young people to start smoking so that we can both prevent smoking and also create policy directed towards cessation. It is estimated that teenagers smoke 1.1 billion packs of cigarettes annually and the eventual health costs from this, added to the subsequent loss of productivity, will amount to over $200 billion per year [3]. Although laws prevent the sales of tobacco products to persons under 18, stronger enforcement of these regulations is necessary to keep cigarettes out of the hands of minors.

A meta-analysis of smoking cessation in teens suggested that, across 48 studies, the probability of successful cessation was improved by 46% when interventions were school- or clinic-based, when there were at least five sessions, and when they used motivation-enhancement, cognitive-behavioral techniques, or social influence approaches [6], [21]. Hence, promoting policy directed at school-based avoidance and cessation programs might be the best strategy. In contrast, a systematic review of randomized controlled trials of smoking prevention interventions at primary care clinics and dentist offices for pediatric patients showed very limited evidence for efficacy of smoking prevention, low efficacy of smoking cessation interventions, and no evidence of long-term effectiveness of either intervention [27]. The controversy in the medical literature about the effectiveness of various tobacco cessation programs in youth suggests that there needs to be more research and larger studies on the methods and results of different tobacco cessation models.

In addition to primary care clinics offering cessation and abstinence counseling, there are other provider sites, including dental offices and emergency departments, which can play a role in influencing the smoking prevalence in this population. Young adults tend to be very aware of their own general and dental appearance, and seem to feel significant appearance-related concerns [28], [29]. Therefore, they may to respond to health campaigns using imagery that depicts stained fingers, wrinkled skin, and the changes of gum disease and stained teeth resulting from continued tobacco use. In emergency departments, there is an additional opportunity to make a difference, for example when youth are presenting with symptoms of diseases such as asthma that may be exacerbated by tobacco abuse. A contact person such as a case manager or social worker in an emergency department could direct such patients into peer counseling programs and make weekly phone calls to see how they were doing with quitting.

KEY POINTS

- The prevalence of smoking among adolescents and young adults is high, especially among white youth. Despite laws preventing the sale of tobacco to minors, children are indirectly targeted by tobacco advertising through the entertainment industry and the use of cartoon characters in advertisements.

- Most adult smokers begin their habit before they are 18 years old. There are a number of significant health impacts of tobacco use on youth.

- Evidence suggests that the best clinical solutions for tobacco cessation in adolescents and young adults include the use of counseling, cognitive-behavioral therapy, and nicotine replacement therapy. However, nicotine products and pharmacological agents are not approved for use in persons under 18 years of age.

- Counteracting tobacco advertising that affect youth and increasing interventions at the level of primary care, dental offices, and emergency departments may be successful health policy initiatives for this patient population.

Health care policy initiatives must also be directed at other significant influences on tobacco abuse in younger populations, such as the entertainment media and movie industry. Changing behaviors and influences in the movie industry could prove to be very difficult due to the constitutional rights of free speech. The counterargument to that would be that there has been a precedent set with the restriction of tobacco advertising on radio and television advertisements and that this is an extension of that restriction. To restrict tobacco smoking in movies that are geared toward children and teens would decrease the "normalization" of tobacco use and thus may decrease the receptiveness of adolescents and young adults to cigarettes. Limiting tobacco advertising in a way to completely exclude cartoon characters additionally seems essential

REFERENCES

[1] Elders MJ, Perry CL, Eriksen MP, Giovino GA. The report of the Surgeon General: Preventing tobacco use among young people. 1994. *American Journal of Public Health.* 84(4):543-547.

[2] Centers for Disease Control and Prevention (2008) Cigarette Use Among High School Students- United States, 1991-2007. *Morbidity and Mortality Weekly Reports (MMWR).* June 27, 2008. 57(25).

[3] Woolf A. Smoking and Nicotine Addiction: A Pediatric Epidemic with Sequelae in Adulthood. *Current Opinion in Pediatrics.* 1997. 9:470-477.

[4] Pbert L, Flint A, Fletcher K, Young M, Drunker S. Effect of a Pediatric Practice Based Smoking Prevention and Cessation Intervention for Adolescents: A Randomized, Controlled Trial. *Pediatrics.* 2008. 121; e738-e747.

[5] Centers for Disease control and Prevention (1998). Selected cigarette smoking initiation and quitting behaviors among high school students – United States 1997. *Morbidity and Mortality Weekly Reports (MMWR).* Vol 47.

[6] McVea, K. Evidence for Clinical Smoking Cessation for Adolescents. *Health Psychology.* 2006. 25(5):558-562.

[7] Hutcheson T, Greiner KA, Ellerbeck E. Understanding smoking cessation in rural communities. Spring 2008 National Rural Health Association.

[8] Pierce JP, Choi WS, Gilpin EA, Farkas AJ, Berry CC. Tobacco Industry Promotion of Cigarettes and Adolescent Smoking. *JAMA.* 1998. 279:511-515.

[9] Waxman H. Tobacco marketing. Profiteering from children [comment]. *JAMA.* Dec. 11, 1991. 266(22):3185-6.

[10] Sargent J, Gibson J, Heatherton TF. Comparing the effects of entertainment media and tobacco marketing on youth smoking. *Tobacco Control.* 2009. 18:47-53.

[11] Dalton MA, Tickle JJ, Sargent JD, Beach ML, Ahrens B, Heatherton TF. The Incidence and Context of Tobacco Use in Popular Movies from 1988 to 1997. *Preventive Medicine.* May 2002. 34(5):516-23.

[12] III.(e) Prohibition on Payments Related to Tobacco Products and Media. *Master Settlement Agreement*, November 23, 1998. Retrieved May 17, 2009 from http://www.naag.org/upload/1032468605_cigmsa.pdf.

[13] National Center for Tobacco-Free Kids. Campaign for Tobacco-Free Kids. Factsheets. Acquired on April 7, 2009 at: http://www.tobaccofreekids.org /research/factsheets/.

[14] Kacirk K, Glantz S. Smoking in Movies in 2000 Exceeded Rates in the 1960s. Letter. *Tobacco Control.* 2001. 10:397-398.

[15] Federal Trade Commission Cigarette Report for 2004-2005. Acquired on May 30, 2009 at: http://www.ftc.gov/reports/tobacco/2007cigarette2004-2005.pdf.

[16] Ling PM, Glantz SA. Why and How the Tobacco Industry Sells Cigarettes to Young Adults: Evidence from Industry Documents. *American Journal of Public Health.* June 2002. 92(6):908-916.

[17] Lovato C, Linn G, Stead LF, Best A. Impact of tobacco advertising and promotion on increasing adolescent smoking behaviors (Review). *Cochrane Database of Systematic Reviews.* 2003. Issue 3. Art. No. CD003439. The Cochrane Collaboration.

[18] King C, Siegel M, Celebucki C, Connolly G. Adolescent Exposure to Cigarette Advertising in Relation to Youth Readership. *JAMA.* February 18, 1998. 279(7):516-520.

[19] Rigotti NA, Moran SE, Wechsler H. US College Students' Exposure to Tobacco Promotions: Prevalence and Association With Tobacco Use. *American Journal of Public Health.* January 2005. 95(1):138-144.

[20] Nicorette Stop Smoking Gum. Frequently asked questions. Retrieved May 24, 2009 from http://www.nicorette.com/Faqs.aspx#21 and http://www.nicorette.com/Nicorette_Know.aspx.

[21] Sussman S, Sun P, Dent CW. A Meta-Analysis of Teen Smoking Cessation. *Health Psychology.* 2006. 25(5):549-557.

[22] Myung S-K, McDonell DD, Kazinets G, Seo HG, Moskowitz JM. Effects of Web- and Computer-Based Smoking Cessation Programs. Meta-analysis of Randomized Controlled Trials. *Archives of Internal Medicine.* May 25, 2009. 169(10):929-937.

[23] Bupropion hydrochloride drug information. Retrieved May 17, 2009 from http://www.fda.gov/cder/drug/infopage/bupropion/default.htm.

[24] Prescribing Information: CHANTIX® (varenicline) Tablets. Dosage and Administration. Retrieved May 17, 2009 from https://www.pfizerpro.com/sites/pfp/pages/product_info/Chantix_pi_dosage _and_adminiadminist.aspx and http://www.pfizer.com/files/products/uspi_chantix.pdf.

[25] Killen JD, Robinson TN, Ammerman S, Hayward C, Rogers J, Stone C, Samuels D, Levin SK, Green S, Schatzbert AF. Randomized Clinical Trial of the Efficacy of Bupropion Combined with Nicotine Patch in the Treatment of Adolescent Smokers. *Journal of Consulting and Clinical Psychology.* 2004. 72(4): 729-735.

[26] Colby SM, Gwaltney CJ. Pharmacotherapy for Adolescent Smoking Cessation. *JAMA.* 2007. 298: 2182-2184.

[27] Christakis D, Garrison M, Ebel B, Wiehe S, Rivara F. Pediatric Smoking Prevention Interventions Delivered by Care Providers: A Systematic Review. *American Journal of Preventative Medicine.* 2003. 25(4). 358-362.

[28] Simis KJ, Koot JM, Verhulst FC, Hovius SER, and The Adolescence Plastic Surgical Research Group. Assessing adolescents and young adults for plastic surgical intervention: pre-surgical appearance ratings and appearance-related burdens as reported by adolescents and young adults, parents and surgeons. *British Journal of Plastic Surgery.* October 2000. 53(7):593-600.

[29] Espeland LV, Stenvik A, Medi L. Concern for dental appearance among young adults in a region with non-specialist orthodontic treatment. *The European Journal of Orthodontics.* 1993. 15(1):17-25.

Chapter 4

TOBACCO DEPENDENCE TREATMENT IN OLDER ADULTS

TOBACCO USE PATTERNS AND PUBLIC HEALTH IMPACT

Older smokers are at greater risks from smoking for many reasons. For one, they have generally smoked for much longer periods of time, with an average tobacco use history of 40 years [1]. The current generation of older adults in the U.S. had smoking rates among the highest of any U.S. generation – in the 1960's, 54% of adult males in this generation were active smokers and 21% were former smokers [2]. This generation also tends to be heavier smokers and its members are more likely to already suffer from a smoking-related illness [1]. Currently, twenty-two percent of adults age 45-65 smoke, but that number decreases drastically to only 9.1% of adults over the age of 65 [3]. One of the reasons for this sharp decline is that mortality is increased in smokers, and users of cigarettes die an average of 13-14 years earlier than nonsmokers [3], [4]. A substantial number of adults in the 45 to 65 year old age range have already started suffering the long-term health consequences of smoking. For those over 65, the health consequences are even greater and persons are dying sooner. Tobacco-related diseases, including heart disease, cancer, and stroke, are the leading cause of disease, disability, and death in the United States [5]. Annually, an estimated 443,000 persons die prematurely in the U.S. from smoking or exposure to second-hand smoke [6]. Another 8.6 million persons have a serious illness caused by smoking [5]. The diseases caused by smoking are numerous and are extensively reviewed elsewhere (see, for example, [1] and [5]).

POPULATION-SPECIFIC BARRIERS TO TREATMENT OF TOBACCO DEPENDENCE

Adults that have been smoking all of their lives are a challenging subset of the population to assist in terms of tobacco cessation. With an average tobacco use history of 40 years and a much longer history of addiction, tobacco dependence may be a harder habit and routine for older adults to break [1], [5]. Older smokers continue to smoke for various reasons, including "habit," for "relaxation," and for "pleasure" [7]. Additionally, older smokers are significantly less likely than younger smokers to believe that smoking harms their health [6], [7]. They also may fear imagined potential health risks from smoking cessation aides, such as nicotine replacement therapy [8], although such worries are often based on inaccurate information. They may also believe that quitting smoking offers no benefit at an advanced age, or that the damage from smoking "has already been done," even though there is robust evidence to suggest that smoking cessation at any age will both prolong life and improve overall quality of life [8]. After one year has passed from quitting tobacco, the added risk of heart disease from smoking is cut almost by 50%, and the risk of stroke, lung disease, and cancer decreases as well [9]. In fact, research suggests that most of the reasons that older adults cite for not wanting to quit tobacco are based on erroneous beliefs [8]. Other barriers to treatment of tobacco addiction in the older age group may overlap with barriers from other population subsets, such as those based on gender or race. In addition, the cost of health care may play a role. For older adults who do have health care insurance such as Medicare, tobacco cessation-related expenses may not always be covered by their plan. If they are living off of a fixed and limited budget from retirement savings or Social Security payments, and particularly if their medication costs are already high, they may not be willing to take on the additional medical- and drug-related costs associated with tobacco cessation.

CLINICAL SOLUTIONS

Motivation to quit seems to be a major factor in assisting older adults with tobacco cessation, and studies suggest that persons with higher levels of medical problems and psychological stress seem to have the greatest desire to quit smoking [10]. Hence, motivational methods may be necessary for those who do not report the same levels of illness and stress. Another important factor in smoking cessation is ensuring that clinicians counsel older patients about quitting. In a study of older adults admitted with acute myocardial infarction, only 40% of these patients had gotten smoking cessation counseling upon discharge from the hospital [4].

Overall, the clinical recommendations for helping older adults quit smoking include the use of counseling and social support, supplemented with nicotine replacement aides and pharmacotherapy. In a recent study of smoking cessation in older adults, nicotine replacement improved cessation rates by four-fold when combined with counseling and ongoing telephone support [12]. Behavior therapy on its own doubles success rates for cessation [10]. Most of the research that focuses on older adults and smoking cessation has been done with nicotine replacement therapy, and there is a relative paucity of research on older adults and newer pharmacologic therapies such as varenicline. Although data are limited, there seems to be no need for dose-adjustment of varenicline in older patients based on age alone, and that the drug may be overall well-tolerated in these patients [13]. Bupropion has been shown to double quit rates and has a low drop-out rate from adverse events [10]. Since various methods are considered to be both efficacious and safe, treatment regimens can be individually tailored to the needs of each patient. However, drug therapies must be used with caution in the older population due to the high incidence of polypharmacy and the potential for adverse inter-drug reactions.

HEALTH POLICY RECOMMENDATIONS

The public health effect of smoking on older adults is staggering. To combat this, ensuring that providers counsel older patients on tobacco cessation is essential. Additionally, for older adults who do have health insurance, mandating that insurers cover pharmacologic agents and services such as behavioral therapy may improve the access of patients to these proven interventions for tobacco cessation. At this time, less than half of insured persons have coverage for counseling services related to tobacco cessation [14].

A strategy to assist older adults who are still in the workforce could be to promote workplace incentives for quitting smoking. A randomized, controlled study in the *New England Journal of Medicine* suggested that this method can be highly successful [15]. In this study, enrollees were provided cessation education and then were randomized to one of two treatment arms. One arm offered a financial incentive of $250 for cessation of smoking within 6 months, and $400 for sustained abstinence for another 6 months. The other treatment arm offered no financial incentive. The group receiving the financial incentive had a statistically-significant, 2- to 3-time higher rate of success than the other group, both in the short term and after 15-18 months of follow-up. The cost of these incentives seems to be reasonably small in comparison to the costs associated with tobacco-related illness, such as lost productivity and increased numbers of sick days. However, incentive programs may have additional expenses, such as random blood testing, which are done to ensure that people who are surreptitiously still smoking do not get the incentives. Further analysis of the savings benefits from an expanded, incentive-based model could be investigated in the future.

KEY POINTS

- Older persons often continue smoking, and cite reasons for not wanting to quit, based on erroneous beliefs that treatment is harmful and quitting offers them little benefit. Missed opportunities by clinicians to counsel older patients on smoking cessation compound the problem. Financial considerations may also play a role.

- Motivation to quit seems to be a major factor in assisting older adults with tobacco cessation, and many tools are available to help these patients quit once they have committed to the idea. Behavioral therapy seems to be beneficial, and pharmacologic agents appear to be safe and well-tolerated. Caution must be used to avoid polypharmacy and drug-drug interactions.

- Mandating that insurers cover pharmacologic agents and services such as behavioral therapy may improve the access of patients to these proven interventions for tobacco cessation. Financial incentives may be another successful health policy strategy.

REFERENCES

[1] Smoking Among Older Adults Fact Sheet. American Lung Association. Retrieved May 24, 2009 from: http://www.lungusa.org/site/c.dvLUK9O0E/b.39862.

[2] Centers for Disease Control and Prevention. National Center for Health Statistics. National Health Interview Survey, 1965-2006. Calculations for 1997-2006 were performed by the American Lung Association Research and Program Services Division using SPSS and SUDAAN software. Retrieved May 24, 2009 from: http://www.lungusa.org/site/c.dvLUK9O0E/b.39862.

[3] U.S. Centers for Disease Control and Prevention (CDC). "Cigarette Smoking Among Adults - United States, 2003." *Morbidity and Mortality Weekly Report (MMWR)*. 54(20):509-513. Retrieved May 24, 2009 from: http://www.cdc.gov/mmwr/preview/mmwrhtml/mm5420a3.htm.

[4] Doolan D, Froelicher E. Effficacy of Smoking Cessation Intervention Among Special Populations. *Nursing Research*. July/August 2006. 55(4S):S29-S37.

[5] United States Center for Disease Control and Prevention. 2009. State Specific Prevalence and Trends in Adult Cigarette Smoking - United States - 1998-2007. *Morbidity and Mortality Weekly Report (MMWR)*. March 13, 2009. 58(09): 221-226.

[6] Rimer BK, Orleans CT, Keintz MK, Cristinzio S, Fleisher L. The older smoker: status, challenges and opportunities for intervention. *Chest*. 1990. 97:547-53.

[7] Donze J, Ruffieux C, Cornuz J. Determinants of smoking and cessation in older women. *Age and Ageing*. 2007. 36:53-57.

[8] Kerr S, Watson H, Tolson D, Lough M, Brown M. Developing Evidence-Based Smoking Cessation Training/Education Initiatives in Partnership with Older People and Health Professionals. Caledonian Nursing and Midwifery Research Centre: Glasgow 2004. Retrieved May 24, 2009 from http://www.lungusa.org/site/c.dvLUK9O0E/b.39862.

[9] Taylor DH, Hasselblad V, Henley J, Thun MD, Sloan FA. Benefits of Smoking Cessation for Longevity. *American Journal of Public Health*. 2002. 92:990-996.

[10] Hughes JR. New treatments for smoking cessation. *CA: A Cancer Journal for Clinicians*. 2000. 50:143.

[11] Sachs-Ericsson N, Schmidt NB, Zvolensky MJ, Mitchell M, Collins N, Blazer DG. Smoking cessation behavior in older adults by race and gender:

The role of health problems and psychological distress. *Nicotine and Tobacco Research.* 2009. 11:433-443.

[12] Tait RJ, Hulse GK, Waterreus A, Flicker L, Lautenschlager NT, Jamrozik K, Almeida OP. Effectiveness of a Smoking Cessation Intervention in Older Adults. *Addiction.* 2006. 102:148-155.

[13] Burstein AH, Fullerton T, Clark DJ, Faessel HM. Pharmacokinetics, Safety, and Tolerability After Single and Multiple Oral Doses of Varenicline in Elderly Smokers. *Journal of Clinical Pharmacology.* 2006. 46: 1234-1240.

[14] McPhilips-Tangum C, Rehm B, Carreon C, Erceg CM, Bocchino C. Addressing Tobacco in Managed Care: Results of the 2003 Survey. *Preventing Chronic Disease.* July 2006. 3(3).

[15] Volpp K, Troxel A, Pauly M. A Randomized, Controlled trial of Financial Incentives for Smoking Cessation. *New England Journal of Medicine.* Feb 12, 2009. 360(7):699-709.

Chapter 5

TOBACCO DEPENDENCE TREATMENT AND PATIENT RACE AND ETHNICITY

TOBACCO USE PATTERNS AND PUBLIC HEALTH IMPACT

The United States is composed of a racially- and ethnically-diverse population. An individual's *race* is an arbitrary and self-designated classification often based on phenotypic characteristics related to a common heredity or descent; *ethnicity* is an arbitrary and self-designated classification often based on common cultural, religious, or linguistic traditions [1]. A person's *culture* may often embody belief systems, attitudes, or behaviors shared by members of groups united by race, ethnicity, or other factors [1], [2]. Cultural factors such as race and ethnicity appear to be important when considering the scope of tobacco abuse and its treatment. Different cultural, racial, and ethnic groups often have a higher prevalence of tobacco dependence than the general population (*see Figure 5.1*), and share unique influences on tobacco-related behavior or even distinctive responses to different tobacco cessation techniques.

For one example, African American smoking rates in 1995 were 31.4% for males and 22.7% for females [3], whereas 21% of the overall United States population smokes tobacco [4]. Data suggest that African Americans may be less dependent on nicotine because they smoke fewer cigarettes per day, but they are also less likely to successfully quit smoking, perhaps due in part to decreased access to preventative health services [3]. Despite these statistics, the prevalence of smoking among African American youth (16.7%) is less than that for white youth (45.4%).

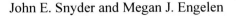

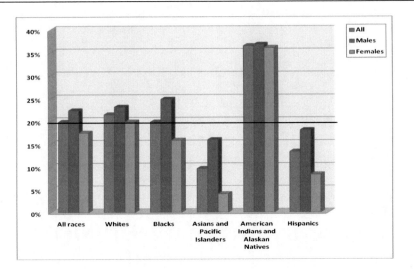

Figure 5.1. By 2007 data, the estimated percentage of adults (persons > 18 years of age) who are current smokers, as differentiated by race and gender. A horizontal bar represents the national current smoking rate for all races and all genders combined (19.8%). Source: U.S. Centers for Disease Control and Prevention (CDC), "Cigarette Smoking Among Adults-United States 2007." Morbidity and Mortality Weekly Report (MMWR). Nov 14, 2008. 57(45): 1221-1226. Acquired on June 4, 2009 at http://www.cdc.gov/mmwr /preview/mmwrhtml/mm5745a2.htm.

African American youth appear to be less likely than whites to believe that cigarettes control their weight, and African American parents seem more likely than their white counterparts to maintain a clear anti-tobacco message for their children [3].

Race may also play a role in the susceptibility to different to diseases caused by tobacco abuse. Even with a lower pack-year history of smoking, African American smokers tend to have a higher incidence of lung cancer than white smokers [5]. Native Hawaiian smokers have a higher rate of lung cancer than whites, Japanese Americans, and Latinos [5]. What predisposes certain racial groups to higher incidences of lung cancer with the same past amount of tobacco exposure is not clear. Environmental factors such as exposure to other lung carcinogens may play a role, and it is possible that there may be an inherent biological difference between races in the ability to metabolize some of the carcinogens and other materials found in cigarettes. It has been shown that even after the same number of cigarettes smoked, African Americans have a higher serum level of cotinine, a metabolite of nicotine that can be used to quantify tobacco exposure, than white or Hispanic smokers [6].

American Indians and Alaska Natives have the highest smoking prevalence rates among all of the racial and ethnic populations in the United States. In American Indian and Alaskan natives, 45.4% of men and 34.2% of females smoke tobacco [3]. Cessation rates are significantly lower in both American Indians and Alaskan natives than in the general population [3]. These communities have had a long history of traditions, passed down through generations, which involve gathering around ceremonial pipes as there is a belief that smoking rituals connect individuals to their spirituality. Smoking has been used in medicinal and healing rituals, in ceremonial and religious practices, as a symbol of peace, and is considered a gift of the earth [7]. Some American Indians may believe that they must continue to smoke, at least traditionally, because it helps them maintain their spirituality and their identity as an Indian [8]. However, there is a great difference between ceremonial smoking and habitual tobacco dependence involving commercial tobacco products. For one, ceremonial smoking typically does not involve inhaling the smoke [7]. Health care providers must understand this difference well in order to be able to influence Native American patients to quit smoking but at the same time to not criticize or interfere with Indian cultural beliefs and traditions.

Asian and Pacific Islanders have an overall lower rate of smoking than the rest of the population, but there is a disparity in the percentage of men versus women smoking. In this group 25.1% of men and only 5.8% of women smoke tobacco [3]. In the Hispanic population, 22.9% of men and 15.1% of Hispanic women smoke tobacco [3]. After adjusting for education level, Hispanics have been found to be more likely than whites to be able to quit smoking [3]. When education is not adjusted for, the overall quit rates are higher for whites than they are for African American and Hispanic populations [3].

POPULATION-SPECIFIC BARRIERS TO TREATMENT OF TOBACCO DEPENDENCE

The 1998 Surgeon General's report on tobacco use in racial and ethnic minority groups shed light on how the tobacco industry has in many ways targeted minority groups with directed marketing campaigns and by other methods of influence [3]. For example, one highlighted study found that three major African-American magazines (*Ebony*, *Jet*, and *Essence)* were paid disproportionately higher amounts than other publications for cigarette advertisements [3]. The tobacco industry has supported African-American cultural events, community organizations, elected political figures, and has made donations to predominantly African-American institutions of higher education and scholarship programs. In regard to the Latino community, the tobacco industry has contributed financial support to primary and secondary schools, colleges, and universities, as well as funded scholarship programs targeting Latinos [3]. Tobacco products have been disproportionately promoted to the Latino community through advertising in community publications and by sponsorship of cultural events. Cigarette brands with names like "*Dorado*" and "*Rio*" have been specifically marketed to the Latino community [3]. The tobacco industry has also focused efforts toward American Indians and Alaskan natives by funding cultural and sporting events, and by developing the "*American Spirit*" brand [3], whose package features both an Indian in a headdress smoking a pipe and other culturally-inspired symbols. In one San Diego study [3], it was found that more tobacco advertising billboards were placed in neighborhoods with higher populations of racial and ethnic minorities, with the highest proportion placed in Asian-American neighborhoods. More tobacco advertising displays were also placed in stores catering to primarily Asian-American clientele.

Access to tobacco products may be greater in areas with higher percentages of minority patients as well. Several studies out of the University of Iowa suggest that this is true [9]. Researchers found that there was a higher density of tobacco outlet stores in counties with a greater percentage of African American residents, and that these counties also had greater prevalence rates of smoking. Areas with the lowest average household incomes and areas with the highest proportions of African American and Latino residents had more than twice as many tobacco outlets along major roadways when compared to wealthier, less diverse areas. The researchers in these studies proposed that tobacco companies may be seeking financial gains by purposefully increasing their presence in financially-disadvantaged areas and in more racially-diverse communities.

Beyond directed marketing, many other barriers clearly exist for racial and ethnic minorities to access health care in general, beyond even that for treatment of tobacco dependence. Although the medical system as a whole may have egalitarian goals, numerous studies have shown that racial minorities are treated differently than their white counterparts for the same medical problems. This issue is beyond that of access to physicians, as even at single institutions, article after article has demonstrated a lack of access to surgeries and procedures, immunizations and other preventive services, radiological studies, and even pain medication by non-white patients [10]. Patients that do not speak or have literacy in English, and especially if they also do not speak Spanish, may also find it difficult to get medical assistance or have interpreter services available to them if they do. Issues can also include fear of coercive treatment [11] and mistrust of the health care system [12].

CLINICAL SOLUTIONS

The use of various techniques for treatment of tobacco dependence in certain racial and ethnic groups has been studied, although not extensively or in large-scale clinical trials. The use of sustained-release bupropion has been specifically examined in African-American patients, with a 21% quit rate observed at 26 weeks. Participants also reported a reduction of depressive symptoms and no associated weight gain [13]. Even though these results are lower than the 30.3% quit rate seen in studies of bupropion in white patients, it still appears to be an important treatment modality for this patient group [14]. Combination treatment with bupropion, nicotine patch, and behavioral counseling shows disproportionately lower success rates among racial and ethnic minorities when compared to white patients [15], but are still overall recommended in nonwhite patients [16] due to a lack of proven alternatives.

In addition to counseling and pharmacological aides, cessation strategies should be catered to individuals and should keep cultural factors in mind. For example, clinical solutions specific to American Indians might include group and individual counseling along with support from the family and community at large [18]. It is also important not to discourage ceremonial use of tobacco because of its significance in the culture of the American Indian. In this population there may also be financial barriers related to the cost and accessibility of nicotine replacement therapy and other pharmacotherapeutic agents [18].

There are a few studies that can help guide specific clinical recommendations in the Latino population, but no large-scale trials that are definitive in nature. A ten-week randomized, double-blind, placebo-controlled trial compared the use of the nicotine patch and counseling with placebo and counseling in Latino patients. It was found that the nicotine patch with counseling improved the abstinence rate, and that the highest abstinence rates were in those Latinos with greater integration into American culture [16], [17]. One of the barriers to addressing tobacco use in the Latino population is that Latinos may perceive smoking as a weakness and not a medical condition that needs to be treated [18]. Studies have suggested that the Latino population has an overall distrust for medical treatments and has a specific aversion to bupropion because of its association with mental illness [18].

The efficacy of varenicline for smoking cessation in minority groups has not been well studied, although in a largely white population it seems to be effective and achieved abstinence rates of around 23% at 52 weeks, compared with bupropion (14.6% abstinence), and placebo (10.3% abstinence) [14]. Although no specific data exists to support or oppose varenicline use in Asian Americans, the drug has been shown to be efficacious and well-tolerated in Asian persons hailing from Taiwan and Japan [19], [20].

HEALTH POLICY RECOMMENDATIONS

Race and ethnicity play an important role in how individuals respond to assistance and clinical advice related to smoking cessation. Policy makers must take into account differences in race and ethnicity when determining solutions for this problem, and not offer blanket recommendations they believe will work for everyone. Numerous studies have demonstrated that demographic subgroups of the general population (based on race, culture, gender, age, and sexual orientation) do not always receive the same diagnostic studies, treatment options, or even preventive care. As tobacco dependence clearly has different characteristics and treatment intricacies among different racial and ethnic groups, it is vital that clinical studies are more inclusive of minorities in the future. Since the health consequences of smoking vary among racial and ethnic groups, this should be highlighted in educational material. There needs to be culturally-sensitive educational materials on quitting smoking that appeal to common beliefs and that doesn't attack or offend a group's identity or spirituality. Language barriers need to be considered for non-English speaking patients, who may benefit from linguistically-appropriate educational materials. Educational programs, pamphlets and other materials written in Spanish or geared toward minority groups can be disseminated through churches or community centers catering to non-white and non-English speaking persons.

Race and ethnicity play an important role in how we must approach challenges in treating tobacco dependence due to cultural barriers. Initiatives such as the youth-oriented 'TheTruth.com' campaign tend to focus their efforts on racial diversity and inclusiveness. A study in the journal *Ethnicity and Health* assessed the impact of the national 'TheTruth.com' antismoking campaign on beliefs, attitudes, and intent to smoke within different racial and ethnic groups [21]. This study suggested that the campaign inspired anti-tobacco beliefs in youth across different races and ethnicities. The campaign tended to have similar impact on both African American and white youth in transmitting a message that cigarette companies lie about the fact that cigarettes are addictive and cause cancer [21]. The impact was slightly less significant in Hispanic and Asian youth.

Similar campaigns geared toward parents and adult smokers may have a broad appeal across racial and ethnic groups, and may help influence individuals who do not normally feel that public health outreach is geared toward their needs.

KEY POINTS

• Different cultural, racial, and ethnic groups have varied prevalence rates of smoking, share unique influences on tobacco-related behavior, are affected by tobacco-related diseases differently, and may even have distinctive responses to different tobacco cessation techniques.

• The use of various techniques for treatment of tobacco dependence in certain racial and ethnic groups has been studied, although not extensively or in large-scale clinical trials. Combination treatment with bupropion, nicotine patch, and behavioral counseling shows disproportionately low success rates among racial and ethnic minorities when compared to white patients, but is still supported due to a lack of proven alternatives. Varenicline may be useful in minority patients, but data specific to these patients is lacking. Culture and language should be considered when tailoring a smoking cessation plan to an individual patient.

• Significant public health policy is needed to address barriers to care for minority groups in general, including but certainly not limited to the treatment of tobacco dependence.

REFERENCES

[1]   *Evidence-Based Medical Ethics: Cases for Practice-Based Learning.* Snyder JE and Gauthier CC. Humana Press, 2008. Page 136.

[2]   culture. (n.d.). *The American Heritage® New Dictionary of Cultural Literacy, Third Edition.* Retrieved May 17, 2009, from Dictionary.com website: http://dictionary1.classic.reference.com/browse/culture

[3]   U.S. Department of Health and Human Services. Tobacco Use Among U.S. Racial/Ethnic Minority Groups—African Americans, American Indians and Alaska Natives, Asian Americans and Pacific Islanders, and Hispanics: A Report of the Surgeon General. Atlanta: U.S. Department of Health and Human Services, Centers for Disease Control and Prevention, 1998 [cited 2007 May 10]. Retrieved May 24, 2009 from: http://www.cdc.gov/tobacco/data_statistics/sgr/sgr_1998/index.htm.

[4]   U.S. Centers for Disease Control and Prevention (CDC), "Cigarette Smoking in Adults – -- United States 2006." *Morbidity and Mortality Weekly Report (MMWR).* November 9, 2007. 56(44):1157-1161. Acquired on June 4, 2009 at: http://www.cdc.gov/mmwr/preview/ mmwrhtml /mm5644a2.htm.

[5]   Haiman C, Daniel S, Wilkens L. Ethnic and Racial Differences in the Smoking-Related Risk of Lung Cancer. *New England Journal of Medicine.* Jan 26, 2006. 354 (4): 333-342.

[6]   Caraballo RS, Giovino GA, Pechacek TF, Mowery PD, Richter PA, Strauss WJ, Sharp DJ, Eriksen MP, Pirkle JL, Maurer KR. Racial and Ethnic Differences in Serum Cotinine Levels of Cigarette Smokers: Third National Health and Nutrition Examination Survey, 1988-1991. 1998. *JAMA.* 280: 135-139.

[7]   Struthers R, Hodge F. Sacred Tobacco Use in Ojibwe Communities. *Journal of Holistic Nursing.* 2004. 22: 209-225.

[8]   Choi WS, Daley CM, James A, Thomas J, Schupbach R, Segraves M, Barnoskie R, Ahluwalia JS. Beliefs and Attitudes Regarding Smoking Cessation Among American Indians: A Pilot Study. *Ethnicity and Disease.* Winter 2006. Vol 16: 35-40.

[9]   UI Health Care News: Week of December 5, 2005. UI Researchers Examine Effect of Race on Smoking, Tobacco Outlet Density. Retrieved May 24, 2009 from http://www.uihealthcare.com/news/ news/2005/12/ 05tobacco. html

[10] Friedman E. Money isn't everything. Nonfinancial barriers to access. *JAMA.* May 18, 1994. 271(19):1535-8.

[11] Hahm HC, Segal SP. Failure to seek health care among the mentally ill. *American Journal of Orthopsychiatry*. 2005 Jan. 75(1):54-62.

[12] Chadda RK, Agarwal V, Singh MC, Raheja D. Help seeking behaviour of psychiatric patients before seeking care at a mental hospital. *International Journal of Social Psychiatry*. 2001. 47(4):71-8.

[13] Ahluwalia JS, McNagny SE, Clark WS. Smoking Cessation among Inner-City African Americans Using the Nicotine Transdermal Patch. *JGIM*. 1998. 13(1):1-8.

[14] Jorenby DE, Hays JT, Rigotti NA, Azoulay S, Watsky EJ, Williams KE, Billing CB, Gong J, Reeves KR. Efficacy of Varenicline, an α4β2 Nicotinic Acetylcholine Receptor Partial Agonist, vs Placebo or Sustained-Release Bupropion for Smoking Cessation. *JAMA*. 2006. 296(1):56-63.

[15] Covey LS, Botello-Harbaum M, Glassman AH, Masmela J, LoDuca C, Salzman V, Fried J. Smoker's response to combination bupropion, nicotine patch, and counseling treatment by race/ethnicity. *Ethnicity and Disease*. 2008 Winter. 18(1):59-64.

[16] Robles GI, Singh-Franco D, Ghin HL. A review of efficacy of smoking-cessation pharmacotherapies in nonwhite populations. *Clinical Therapeutics*. 2008 May. 30(5):800-812.

[17] Leischow SJ, Hill A, Cook G. The Effects of Transdermal Nicotine for the Treatment of Hispanic Smokers. *American Journal of Health Behavior*. 1996. 20(5): 304-311.

[18] Levinson AH, Borrayo EA, Espinoza P, Flores ET, Perez-Stable EJ. An Exploration of Latino Smokers and the Use of Pharmaceutical Aids. *American Journal of Preventive Medicine*. 2006. 31(2):167-171.

[19] Nakamura M, Oshima A, Fujimoto Y, Maruyama N, Ishibashi T, Reeves KR. Efficacy and tolerability of varenicline, an α4β2 nicotinic acetylcholine receptor partial agonist, in a 12-week, randomized, placebo-controlled, dose-response study with 40-week follow-up for smoking cessation in Japanese smokers. *Clinical Therapeutics*. 2007 Jun. 29(6):1040-56.

[20] Tsai ST, Cho HJ, Cheng HS, Kim CH, Hsueh KC, Billing CB, Williams KE. A randomized, placebo-controlled trial of varenicline, a selective α4β2 nicotinic acetylcholine receptor partial agonist, as a new therapy for smoking cessation in Asian smokers. *Clinical Therapeutics*. 2007 Jun. 29(6):1027-39.

[21] Cowell A, Farrelly MC, Chou R, Vallone DM. Assessing the impact of the national 'truth' antismoking campaign on beliefs, attitudes, and intent to smoke by race/ethnicity. *Ethnicity and Health*. 2009 Feb. 14(1):75-91.

Chapter 6

TOBACCO DEPENDENCE TREATMENT AND PATIENT SEXUAL ORIENTATION

TOBACCO USE PATTERNS AND PUBLIC HEALTH IMPACT

Persons who self-identify as lesbian, gay, bisexual, or transgendered (LGBT) compose a large and diverse cultural group [1]. LGBT persons cannot be uniformly characterized, as much as members of any cultural group can be, and factors such as racial and ethnic associations may contribute to an individual's cultural identity. Nonetheless, LGBT persons may share certain cultural bonds and belief systems due to similar sociocultural experiences. LGBT persons are also generally united in the idea that their gender identity and sexual orientation are innate and cannot be changed.

LGBT persons, as a cultural group, may have unique risks for certain disease conditions that are different than those of the general population (see, for example, [2] through [10]), and these risks may be based on both heritable and cultural factors. Physicians must remain attentive to and screen for disease processes that are highly prevalent amongst individuals of cultural groups within their patient population. One example is the disproportionately increased rate of smoking observed in the gay, lesbian, and bisexual communities. The prevalence rate of tobacco use among LGBT persons has been quoted as high as 50% in some studies, as compared with 21% of the general population [11]. The public health impact of this high rate of smoking is not yet known, as this has not been a widely published area of research [1], [12], [13]. However, it is likely that there are several resulting and serious health consequences from this degree of tobacco exposure.

POPULATION-SPECIFIC BARRIERS TO TREATMENT OF TOBACCO DEPENDENCE

It has been proposed that several barriers to accessing health care in general exist for LGBT patients, and that these negatively affect both acute medical care and preventive services [14]. A major identified barrier has been that of bias on the part of health care providers, and the resulting fear of discriminatory treatment on the part of patients. Improving access of LGBT patients to high quality health care will require active education of providers to assist in overcoming biases. Providing a safe and accepting health care environment will allow for more opportunities to address health issues, such as tobacco cessation, with LGBT patients.

One of the identifiable barriers to the treatment of tobacco dependence in LGBT persons is that the tobacco industry specifically targets this population in advertising [15]. There is a significant amount of both commercial and noncommercial imagery and text relating to tobacco and smoking in gay, lesbian, and bisexual magazines and newspapers, which tend to shed a positive light on smoking or associate tobacco use with celebrities [16]. Some media marketing is targeted toward LGBT youth smokers [13]. The effect of this is a relative normalization of tobacco use in this population. Tobacco companies have also sponsored LGBT events [17], offered disproportionately high amounts of free product samples to LGBT persons [18], and in 1990, Philip Morris gained LGBT support by pledging to donate large sums of money in the fight against HIV/AIDS [12]. The end result is that tobacco companies have been to some degree welcomed by the LGBT population, being touted for having a strong commitment to diversity and overall support for the LBGT community.

CLINICAL SOLUTIONS

Clinical recommendations for patients in the lesbian, gay, bisexual, and transgendered population are similar as to those in the general population, and include the use of nicotine replacement therapy, counseling, and pharmacotherapeutic agents such as bupropion and varenicline. However, in research involving bupropion and varenicline, there have not been specific studies looking at this target subpopulation. In general, there needs to be more research directed at tobacco cessation in this high-risk group.

One of the important factors to emphasize in the LGBT population is the importance of peer support. A pilot study investigating smoking cessation in gay men found that, with ongoing peer support and nicotine replacement therapy, there was a 76% rate of abstinence after 7 weeks [19]. This success rate is far higher than the overall national data for this combined approach, which has up to a 53% success rate. Although studies in the LGBT population are still limited by number and scope, the available information to date suggests that this population can be quite successful in tobacco cessation with peer support and nicotine replacement therapy.

HEALTH POLICY RECOMMENDATIONS

Most importantly, improving overall access to medical care to LGBT persons needs to be a public health priority. This requires providing a safe and accepting environment for LGBT patients so that access to care and preventive services, including tobacco cessation, will increase. Educational material on providing welcoming care for the LGBT patient is available from many sources, including the website for the Gay and Lesbian Medical Association (*http://www.glma.org*).

Focusing on the differences in exposure to tobacco products and marketing in the LGBT population can give direction of creating policy and strategies for tobacco cessation. Policy must be directed at both limiting the tobacco industry's targeting of this cultural group and also by counter-advertising in directed media, publications, and events. In addition, focus should be on educating influential leaders in the gay, lesbian, bisexual, and transgendered community to actively oppose use of tobacco advertising in print media that is directed towards that population. Historically, LGBT persons have been successfully able to organize around a cause when they feel that they have been exploited [10]. Hence, a successful approach may be to improve information flow to LGBT persons on how the tobacco companies are exploiting them by directly marketing a product to them which is known to cause one in five deaths in this country each year [20]. This may help decrease the normalization of tobacco use that is seen with overwhelming prevalence in directed media. The 'Truth.com' campaign attempted to transmit the message, particularly to youth from diverse racial and ethnic backgrounds, that tobacco companies lie about the fact that cigarettes are addictive and cause cancer [21]. Given the particularly high prevalence rate of smoking in LGBT persons, and the significant media targeting to young and adult LGBT persons, a similar campaign could be geared toward this patient subpopulation. Public health efforts directed toward the LGBT community may strengthen goodwill within this population of people who do not normally feel that their needs are adequately respected and addressed by society and government.

KEY POINTS

• The prevalence rate of tobacco use among LGBT persons has been quoted as high as 50% in some studies; hence it is likely that this population is at high risk for the serious health consequences of tobacco exposure. The true impact is not known as public health studies for this patient population are lacking.

• Clinical recommendations for LGBT patients include the use of nicotine replacement therapy, counseling, and pharmacotherapeutic agents such as bupropion and varenicline. Preliminary data suggests that peer support, combined with nicotine replacement therapy, appears to have a very high rate of success.

• Providing a safe and accepting health care environment will allow for more opportunities to address health issues, such as tobacco cessation, with LGBT patients. Public health efforts directed toward the LGBT community may strengthen goodwill within this population.

REFERENCES

[1] Snyder JE. A Review and Analysis of Medical Publications about LGBT Patients. Unpublished data. Submitted to the *Journal of Homosexuality*, under review, 2010.

[2] Brandenburg DL, Matthews AK, Johnson TP, Hughes TL. Breast cancer risk and screening: a comparison of lesbian and heterosexual women. *Women Health*. 2007. 45(4):109-30.

[3] Case P, Austin SB, Hunter DJ et al. Sexual orientation, health risk factors, and physical functioning in the Nurses' Health Study II. *Journal of Women's Health (Larchmont, N.Y.)*. 2004 Nov. 13(9):1033-47.

[4] Chin-Hong PV, Vittinghoff E, Cranston RD, et al. Age-related prevalence of anal cancer precursors in homosexual men: the EXPLORE study. *Journal of the National Cancer Institute*. 2005 Jun 15. 97(12):896-905.

[5] Daling JR, Weiss NS, Hislop G, Maden C, Coates RJ, Sherman KJ, Ashley RL, Beagrie M, Ryan JA, Corey L. Sexual practices, sexually transmited diseases, and the incidence of anal cancer. *New England Journal of Medicine*. 1987. 317:973–7.

[6] Denenberg R. Report on lesbian health. *Women's Health Issues*. 1995. 5(2):181–91.

[7] Dibble SL, Roberts SA, Robertson PA, Paul SM. Risk factors for ovarian cancer: lesbian and heterosexual women. *Oncology Nursing Forum*. 2002 Jan-Feb. 29(1):E1-7.

[8] Goldstone SE, Hundert JS, Huyett JW. Infrared coagulator ablation of high-grade anal squamous intraepithelial lesions in HIV-negative males who have sex with males. *Diseases of the Colon and Rectum*. 2007 May. 50(5):565-75.

[9] Lesbian Health Fact Sheet. Office on Women's Health, U.S. Department of Health and Human Services. Retrieved May 22, 2008 from http://www.glma.org/_data/n_0001/resources/live/lesbian1.pdf.

[10] Robertson P, Schacter J. Failure to identify venereal disease in a lesbian population. *Sexually Transmitted Diseases*. 1981. 8(2):75–6.

[11] U.S. Centers for Disease Control and Prevention (CDC), "Cigarette Smoking in Adults -- United States 2006." *Morbidity and Mortality Weekly Report (MMWR)*. November 9, 2007. 56(44):1157-1161. Acquired on June 4, 2009 at: http://www.cdc.gov/mmwr/preview/mmwrhtml/mm5644a2.htm.

[12] Stevens P, Carlson L, Hinman J. An Analysis of Tobacco Industry Marketing to Lesbian, Gay, Bisexual, and Transgender Populations:

Strategies for Mainstream Tobacco Control and Prevention. *Health Promotion Practice*. July 2004. 5(3) (Supplement): S129-S134.

[13] Washington HA. Burning Love: Big Tobacco Takes Aim at LGBT Youth. *American Journal of Public Health*. July 2002. 92(7):1086-1095.

[14] Dean L, Meyer IH, Robinson K, Sell RL, Sember R, Silenzio VMB, Bowen DJ, Bradford J, Rothblum E, White J, Dunn P, Lawrence A, Wolfe D, Xavier J. Lesbian, Gay, Bisexual, and Transgender Health: Findings and Concerns. *JGLMA: Journal of the Gay and Lesbian Medical Association*. 2000. 4(3):101-151.

[15] Doolan D, Froelicher E. Effficacy of Smoking Cessation Intervention Among Special Populations. *Nursing Research*. July/August 2006. 55(4S):S29-S37.

[16] United States Center for Disease Control and Prevention. 2009. State Specific Prevalence and Trends in Adult Cigarette Smoking - United States - 1998-2007. *Morbidity and Mortality Weekly Report (MMWR)*. March 13, 2009. 58(09): 221-226.

[17] Smith EA, Malone RE. The Outing of Philip Morris: Advertising Tobacco to Gay Men. *American Journal of Public Health*. June 2003. 93(6):988-993.

[18] Dilley JA, Spigner C, Boysun MJ, Dent CW, Pizacani BA. Does tobacco industry marketing excessively impact lesbian, gay and bisexual communities? *Tobacco Control*. 2008. 17:385-390.

[19] Harding R, Bensley J, Corrigan N. Targeting Smoking Cessation to High Prevalence Communities: Outcomes from a Pilot Intervention for Gay Men. *BMC Public Health*. 2004. 4:43.

[20] U.S. Centers for Disease Control and Prevention (CDC), " Women and smoking: A Report of the Surgeon General. Chapter 5: Efforts to reduce tobacco use among women." *Morbidity and Mortality Weekly Report (MMWR)*. August 30, 2002. 51(RR12):1-30. Acquired on June 4, 2009 at: http://www.cdc.gov/mmwr/preview/mmwrhtml/rr5112a4.htm.

[21] Cowell A, Farrelly MC, Chou R, Vallone DM. Assessing the impact of the national 'truth' antismoking campaign on beliefs, attitudes, and intent to smoke by race/ethnicity. *Ethnicity and Health*. 2009 Feb. 14(1):75-91.

Chapter 7

TOBACCO DEPENDENCE TREATMENT AND PATIENT NATIVE LANGUAGE

TOBACCO USE PATTERNS AND PUBLIC HEALTH IMPACT

Language may be a key shared element by the people within a cultural group. And although all non-English speakers as a whole do not share a unified cultural bond, their native languages create similar demographic and systematic barriers for them, and these barriers place them at a strong disadvantage for maneuvering the increasingly complex U.S. health care system. Patients that do not speak or have literacy in English, and especially if they also do not speak Spanish, may find it difficult to obtain medical assistance or have interpreter services available to them if they do. According to data from the U.S. Census Bureau, in the year 2000, 47 million U.S. residents – nearly one in five persons – speak a language other than English at home [1]. This was a 46% increase from 1990 data, and the number of Spanish speakers within that group rose by 62% to a total of 28.1 million persons. Of the Hispanic population in the United States, 41% speak only Spanish or have limited proficiency in English [2]. There are additionally many persons in the U.S. who don't speak English or Spanish. Two million persons identified by the Census Bureau in 2000 spoke Chinese, the third most common language from the survey data [1].

Data on the public health impact of smoking in non-English speakers have not been previously well-characterized. The largest group of non-English speakers has Spanish as their native language, and greater data is available on persons self-identifying with Hispanic ethnicity (hence, Latino persons). Limited data analyzed from the 2001 The California Health Interview Survey (CHIS) suggests that smoking prevalence rates among Californian Asian Americans differs on the basis of ethnic origin, gender, and level of English proficiency [3]. In that study, Asian men who had high English proficiency were less likely to be smokers than those with lower English proficiency, but the opposite effect was seen among Asian women. Clearly, much more needs to be understood on the public health impact that native language has on health and health care disparities, including that of tobacco dependence.

POPULATION-SPECIFIC BARRIERS TO TREATMENT OF TOBACCO DEPENDENCE

With English as the official language in the United States, most health care information is primarily available in that language. Although a great deal of services may be available to patients in English and Spanish, access to these services is not universal, and there are a large number of persons in the U.S. who speak neither English nor Spanish. Some of the barriers to receiving health care services in patients with non-English native languages are the same barriers that are seen in other cultural groups, such as those united by race or gender. Low socioeconomic status can also play a significant role. In major U.S. cities such as New York and Los Angeles, the most powerful predictor of poverty and hardship, including low income, lacking health insurance, and food insecurity, is having limited English skills [4]. In one study of race, ethnicity, and native language and their effects on health care access for insured patients [5], data suggested that disparities in care for Hispanic patients were largely explained by differences in English proficiency. Spanish-speakers in that study were significantly less likely to have had a physician visit, mental health visit, or influenza vaccination than non-Hispanic white patients. Other studies, however, have conflicting results to this. One such study suggested that although the majority of U.S. Hispanics speak English at home or comfortably in society, they were at increased risk for not receiving recommended health care services whether they were comfortable in speaking English or not [5]. Thus, the issue remains complex and unclear. It seems than other cultural characteristics of non-English speaking persons, in addition to native tongue, may play a significant role in access to health care.

CLINICAL SOLUTIONS

One of the major barriers to treatment of patients with a native language other than English is communication difficulty. To treat tobacco use effectively, there must be good communication between the provider and patient, both in terms of counseling and in instructions for using nicotine replacement therapy or medications such as varenicline and bupropion. Data on the efficacy of pharmacotherapeutic agents in non-English speakers is not available. Therefore, clinical solutions would be the same for non-English speakers as it would be in the general population. These would include treating patients with counseling, nicotine replacement therapy, and pharmacotherapeutic agents. The caveat is that there must be culturally-sensitive education for patients in their native language, and that takes other aspects of culture (such as race and gender) into consideration. It would also be ideal to have community support groups with the same native language to help with peer counseling for smoking cessation. A trial through the National Cancer Institute's Cancer Information Service has also shown that one way to work around the language barrier in Spanish-speaking smokers is to provide counseling services over the phone in Spanish [2]. As evidence also supports the clinical benefit of computer- and internet-based smoking cessation programs [6], this modality could be easily adapted to languages other than English.

HEALTH POLICY RECOMMENDATIONS

Increasing access to interpreter services at health care centers would be an important start in providing improved outreach to non-English-speaking patients. Data suggest that this intervention alone can significantly decrease disparities for non-English-speaking patients in clinical service use, screening tests, and preventive services such as immunization [7]. Training initiatives for bilingual social workers and other persons capable of smoking cessation counseling would also be beneficial. Educational programs using pamphlets and books written in Spanish and other languages can be not only made available at physician's offices and health care clinics, but can also be disseminated through churches and community centers catering to non-English speaking communities. Informing health care providers about counseling services available in other languages, such as telephone quit lines, may also increase their utilization.

KEY POINTS

• Nearly one in five persons speaks a language other than English at home. Other cultural characteristics of non-English speaking persons, in addition to native tongue, may both play a significant role in access to health care and smoking cessation services.

• Clinical solutions for treatment of tobacco dependence are the same for non-English speakers as in the general population, and include counseling, nicotine replacement therapy, and use of pharmacotherapeutic agents. Patient education must be culturally-sensitive and offered, if possible, in a patient's native language. Other aspects of culture (such as race and gender) should be taken into consideration.

• Increasing access to interpreter services, improving educational materials (using pamphlets and books written in Spanish and other languages) and programs, and using greater community outreach may be effective public health strategies for non-English speakers.

REFERENCES

[1] Bergman M. Nearly 1-in-5 Speak a Foreign Language at Home; Most Also Speak English 'Very Well,' Census Bureau Reports. Public Information Office, U.S. Census Bureau, U.S. Department of Commerce. Retrieved May 25, 2009 from http://www.census.gov/Press-Release/www/releases/ archives/ census_2000/001406.html.

[2] Wetter D, Mazas C, Daza P, Nguyen L, Fouladi R, Li Y, Cofta-Woerpel L. Reaching and Treating Spanish-Speaking Smokers Through the National Cancer Center Institute's Cancer Information Service: A Randomized Controlled Trial. *Cancer.* 2007 Jan 15. 109(2 Suppl) 406-413.

[3] Cheng EM, Chen A, Cunningham W. Primary Language and Receipt of Recommended Health Care Among Hispanics in the United States. *JGIM.* 2007 November. 22(Suppl 2): 283–288.

[4] Fix M, Capps R. "Immigrant Well-Being in New York and Los Angeles," Policy Brief No. 1 in series "Immigrant Families and Workers: Facts and Perspectives." Aug. 7, 2003. Retrieved May 25, 2009 from http://www.urban.org/url.cfm?ID=310566.

[5] Fiscella K, Franks P, Doescher MP, Saver BG. Disparities in Health Care by Race, Ethnicity, and Language Among the Insured: Findings From a National Sample. *Medical Care.* January 2002. 40(1):52-59.

[6] Myung S-K, McDonell DD, Kazinets G, Seo HG, Moskowitz JM. Effects of Web- and Computer-Based Smoking Cessation Programs. Meta-analysis of Randomized Controlled Trials. *Archives of Internal Medicine.* May 25, 2009. 169(10):929-937.

[7] Jacobs EA, Lauderdale DS, Meltzer D, Shorey JM, Levinson W, Thisted RA. Impact of interpreter services on delivery of health care to limited-English-proficient patients. *Journal of General Internal Medicine.* 2001. 16:468-74.

Chapter 8

TOBACCO DEPENDENCE TREATMENT AND CULTURAL BARRIERS: CONCLUSIONS

Culture plays an important role in the management of tobacco dependence. Different cultural groups are individually targeted by tobacco industry marketing. Addiction to nicotine and response to pharmacotherapeutic agents may be different based on a person's cultural background, although research in these areas has been limited. Due to various barriers, different cultural groups have unequal access to treatment, medications, support, and other health care resources. As a result, the prevalence of smoking and tobacco-related diseases, as well as the overall burden of these diseases, is higher within these patient populations.

The solutions for these problems lie in the hands of three different parties. The health care provider must be willing and able to offer culturally-competent care and treatment recommendations to assist individual patients with tobacco cessation. The policy-maker must assist in breaking down barriers to fair and equitable access within the health care system. And researchers need to consider the unique qualities and needs of various cultural groups when conducting studies on tobacco dependence, and further assess the efficacy of various interventions within these groups.

Hundreds of thousands of persons die annually in the U.S. alone from tobacco-related diseases, resulting in billions of dollars spent in yearly health care costs. Tobacco is a leading cause of death and disability, and yet tobacco dependence is a completely preventable and treatable disease. The cost-per-life-year saved for treatment is negligible compared to that of other common diseases. In order to ensure that the health care provider, the policy maker, and the researcher all coordinate their efforts to make the greatest impact on this crisis, public health leaders must take charge and champion this cause. Education can help prevent smoking initiation in youth and to motivate all smokers to quit. Learning opportunities will also strengthen providers' efforts and abilities to assist their patients in cessation. Medications and support resources can be made available at low- to no-cost for those who need them. And public smoking bans can be imposed across the nation. Through such efforts, significant strides can be made to help persons from all cultural backgrounds achieve better opportunities for improved health and well-being.

PART II.
SYSTEMATIC BARRIERS
TO TREATING TOBACCO DEPENDENCE

SYSTEMATIC BARRIERS TO TREATING TOBACCO DEPENDENCE – INTRODUCTION

Tobacco dependence is a chronic illness with severe, adverse implications on the smoker's health and well-being. Additionally, the public health impact of tobacco-related illness is staggering. The highly preventable nature of this disease spectrum makes smoking cessation a major public health priority. Health care providers must address smoking on the level of the individual patient, while policy makers and government leaders need to address the issue on the population level. To make the biggest impact on tobacco-related disease, we must better understand the influences that encourage smoking and the barriers to successful cessation in the most at-risk patient populations.

Patients in certain socioeconomic and demographic groups are uniquely vulnerable to tobacco dependence for many reasons. Barriers within the health care system at-large play a significant role, as do geographic and economic factors, insurance status, ability to read, and the presence of underlying mental illness. Other factors include directed and aggressive tobacco industry marketing techniques, barriers to accessing health care providers who provide treatment for tobacco dependence, inequitable access to pharmacological treatment options, and a limited availability of or access to support resources. In the second part of this book, we first present an evidence-based approach for providers that helps identify the most at-risk patients. We then offer specific clinical strategies for approaching tobacco cessation which are proven to be the most effective in overcoming these systematic barriers. Lastly, we propose a number of health policy recommendations which can assist with breaking down barriers to care for each patient group and result in more effective cessation programs on the population level.

Chapter 9

TOBACCO DEPENDENCE TREATMENT AND SYSTEMATIC BARRIERS

Each year, 8 million Americans suffer from tobacco-related diseases and 400,000 Americans die as a result – more than from any other cause [1], [2]. There are $96.7 billion in annual health care costs associated with tobacco use, $38 billion of which are funded by U.S. taxpayer dollars [3]. A disproportionate burden of these illnesses is carried by low-income and uninsured persons, who have decreased access to health care services. The estimated cost-per-life-year saved from tobacco cessation ranges from $2,300-4,200 [4]. However, although the majority of all smokers express a desire to quit (around 70%), only about 8% of all smokers who attempt to quit each year are successful [5].

The health care provider's office provides the perfect opportunity for the initiation of discussions with an individual about quitting smoking. However, clinicians must do a better job in identifying which patients are smokers, offering assistance and tools for tobacco cessation, and following through with counseling at subsequent appointments. Clinical experience has revealed that most patients will not initiate a discussion about their tobacco use or smoking habits unless their provider prompts them. Therefore there are many guidelines, including from the Agency for Health Care Policy and Research, which suggest that clinicians should identify a patient's smoking status and counsel them on smoking cessation at each visit [6]. In a national survey of physicians, 62% of specialists determined smoking status during clinical visits, compared to 67% of primary care physicians [6]. Even though most physicians do ask their patients if they are smoking, studies also suggest that less than 40% of physicians actually provide them with assistance in quitting [7]. The percent of clinical visits that included time spent on smoking counseling was only 15% among specialists and 33% among primary care providers [6].

The disconnect between asking a patient about smoking and actually providing them with counseling and assistance with smoking cessation has been studied, and there are many barriers that affect this trend. In one study, clinicians agreed that barriers included having an inadequate amount of time, patients being unready to quit, inadequate patient resources for both the underserved and insured, inadequate provider resources (educational materials and staff), and inadequate clinical skills to deal with tobacco cessation [8]. One study on tobacco cessation counseling showed that providers are more likely to address smoking cessation in patients with diseases and diagnoses related to smoking such as COPD, alcohol and drug abuse, peptic ulcer disease, respiratory infections, asthma, and heart disease [6]. They are also more likely to discuss cessation with patients that are sicker, rather than healthy patients [9]. Even though it is important to address smoking cessation in patients with specific tobacco-related diseases, care needs to be taken that smoking cessation be addressed in all patient encounters. Smoking cessation is becoming an increasingly emphasized part of medical training curricula and should be equally emphasized in continuing medical education programs.

Other factors play a role as well. Persons with comorbid psychiatric illnesses are more likely to be smokers and statistically tend to have less success in quitting. Tobacco dependence rates are also higher within specific low-income groups, such as the rural and urban poor. There is also often decreased access to preventative health care in these areas, as well as a greater peer influence component that affects an individual's smoking habits. Higher rates of tobacco dependence within patient subpopulations put patients in those groups at higher risk for the health consequences associated with smoking.

In addition to varied smoking prevalence rates, there is also a discrepancy seen in the frequency of tobacco cessation counseling done by physicians to patients in different sociocultural subpopulations. For example, women, ethnic minorities, persons with Medicaid, and patients who are uninsured are all less likely to receive appropriate tobacco counseling and cessation services by physicians [10]. Due to the health consequences of smoking, those in the medical profession and in the public health field need to work harder to augment the number of people who try and successfully quit smoking. But in order to accomplish this task, we must better understand the factors associated with smoking in specific target patient populations, as well as the barriers of these patients to successfully quit smoking.

REFERENCES

[1]   U.S. Centers for Disease Control and Prevention (CDC), "Annual Smoking-Attributable Mortality, Years of Potential Life Lost, and Economic Costs—United States 1997-2001." *Morbidity and Mortality Weekly Report (MMWR).* July 1, 2005. 54(25):625-628. Acquired on May 30, 2009 at: http://www.cdc.gov/mmwr/preview/mmwrhtml/mm5425a1.htm.

[2]   U.S. Centers for Disease Control and Prevention (CDC), "Cigarette smoking Attributable Morbidity – United States, 2000," *Morbidity and Mortality Weekly Report (MMWR).* September 5, 2003. 52(35): 842-844. Acquired on May 30, 2009 at: http://www.cdc.gov/mmwr/PDF/wk/mm5235.pdf.

[3]   National Center for Tobacco-Free Kids. Campaign for Tobacco-Free Kids. Factsheets. Acquired on April 7, 2009 at: http://www.tobaccofreekids.org/research/factsheets/.

[4]   Warner KE, Mendez D, Smith DG. The Financial Implications of Coverage of Smoking Cessation Treatment by Managed Care Organizations. 2004. Inquiry 41 (1): 57-69.

[5]   Gollust S, Schroeder S, Warner K. Helping Smokers Quit: Understanding the Barriers to Utilization of Smoking Cessation Services. *The Milbank Quarterly.* 2008. 86(4): 601-627.

[6]   Thorndike A, Rigotti N, Stafford R, Singer D. National Patterns in the Treatment of Smokers by Physicians. *JAMA.* 1998. 279 (8):604-608.

[7]   Association of American Medical Colleges (AAMC). Physician Behavior and Practice Patterns Related to Smoking Cessation. A Report Prepared for the American Legacy Foundation by the Association of Medical Colleges. May 17, 2007. Acquired on June 2, 2009 at: http://www.americanlegacy.org/261.aspx.

[8]   Blumenthal DS. Barriers to the Provision of Smoking Cessation Services Reported by Clinicians in Underserved Communities. *Journal of the American Board of Family Medicine.* 2007. 20:272-279.

[9]   Houston TK, Scarinci IC, Person SD, Greene PG. Patient Smoking Cessation Advice by Health Care Providers: The Role of Ethnicity, Socioeconomic Status, and Health. *American Journal of Public Health.* 2005. 95(6):1056-61.

[10]   Report of the Surgeon General on Tobacco Use Among US Racial/Ethnic Minority Groups. Washington DC: US Department of Health and Human Services 1998.

Chapter 10

TOBACCO DEPENDENCE TREATMENT
IN THE URBAN POOR

TOBACCO USE PATTERNS AND PUBLIC HEALTH IMPACT

Urban poverty has been argued to be tantamount to a situation of exclusion from the basic rights of citizenship – including exclusion from having a political voice, quality housing and education, safety, transportation, goods and services, legal protection, and opportunities for income and self-betterment [1], [2]. The health care impact of living in low-income urban settings is apparent in many disease processes, such as the higher rates observed for cardiovascular heart disease (CHD) [3]. Smoking among the urban poor is of particular concern because smokers have a higher rate of CHD and hypertension, hence socioeconomic status may put individuals in this population at particularly high risk for the adverse effects of smoking [3]. There are higher overall rates of high cholesterol, hypertension, physical inactivity, and poor diet in these communities [4]. Overall, the urban poor tend also to have a disproportionably high rate of tobacco abuse [5]. In one study of the urban poor in Houston, the nation's 4th largest city, smoking prevalence rates were measured to be 53% among white residents, 42% among black residents, and 24% in the Hispanic population [3]. Residents of public housing also have higher reported rates of tobacco abuse [5].

POPULATION-SPECIFIC BARRIERS TO TREATMENT OF TOBACCO DEPENDENCE

Access to health care in the urban poor is a critical public health issue, with large systematic barriers at play. In urban populations where the average household income is below $15,000, the rate of uninsured can be as high as 75% [6]. Nearly half of persons in these conditions, even if they have access to public health clinics, may avoid health services completely due to financial concerns [6]. Even among the urban poor and near-poor who are privately insured, the cost of co-pays and deductibles limits their usage of health care services [7].

The difference in smoking prevalence rates in low socioeconomic urban areas appears to be due to a greater smoking initiation rate and a lower quit rate [3]. This may be due to the increased targeting of tobacco company advertising in these areas, the social structure that supports an environment of smoking, and the increased stress of living in these environments. The poor in general are targeted by the tobacco companies by some of their biggest promotional offers, including by offering cheaper cigarettes, multi-pack discounts, and coupons to make cigarettes more affordable [8]. Tobacco companies spent $13.11 billion (U.S.) in 2005 on advertising and promotion, with the largest amount of those expenditures being discounts to retailers to decrease the price of tobacco [9]. It has been observed that stores actively participating in tobacco company incentive programs often have lower prices for cigarettes and are more likely to feature cigarettes and advertising materials in a prominent manner [10]. Discounts target the low socioeconomic class as this population is likely to be highly sensitive to price increases and taxing on cigarettes.

The main barriers to tobacco cessation in underserved communities appear to be lack of time to undertake the cessation process, patients not feeling ready to quit smoking, inadequate access to patient resources, inadequate provider resources that are available, and inadequate clinical skills of providers that offer cessation [11]. Additionally, patients without insurance are more likely to be unable to afford the pharmacological options for helping with smoking cessation, such as nicotine replacement therapy, bupropion, and varenicline. Patients with low income may have a lesser willingness to sacrifice the money that they would be paying for cigarettes for medications to help them quit. Surveyed providers for this population feel that there are not enough community resources that they can refer their patients to for help, and that there is inadequate time to do all of the necessary tobacco cessation counseling required in a 15 minute office visit [11]. There may also be frustration among providers serving patient populations with low quit rates, with the feeling that their efforts in trying to get patients to quit smoking are not often enough successful. Yet persistence, including continued discussion about tobacco cessation at every single office visit, may eventually lead to more successful quit rates for patients.

CLINICAL SOLUTIONS

Clinical solutions for the treatment of tobacco dependence are the same for the urban poor as in the general population, and include counseling and peer support, nicotine replacement therapy, and the use of pharmacotherapeutic agents such as bupropion and varenicline. However, barriers to care for the urban poor must be considered when initiating a tobacco cessation plan. Patients may not have time outside of work to participate in individual or group quit programs. Patients also may be unable to afford prescribed medications or nicotine replacement therapy.

In research involving varenicline and bupropion, there have not been specific studies looking at this target subpopulation. In general, there needs to be more research directed at tobacco cessation in this high-risk group that carries such a high burden of disease related to tobacco use. One study in urban, low-income, African American patients examined the use of nicotine replacement therapy (via the patch) in combination with counseling versus placebo and counseling, and found that the short-term quit rates are significantly improved from the use of nicotine replacement (21.5% versus 13.7% respectively) [12]. In another study of low-income, African American, inner-city smokers, there was an increased quit rate associated with culturally-sensitive self-help tobacco cessation literature combined with a single phone contact [13]. Computer- and internet-based smoking cessation programs may be of benefit as well [14].

HEALTH POLICY RECOMMENDATIONS

The poor are targeted by tobacco company promotions and discounts, which make cigarettes more affordable for this population [8]. One of the ways to counteract such incentives and decrease tobacco dependence is to create policy to increase tobacco taxation. This approach may be of particular benefit to lower socioeconomic groups.

KEY POINTS

- Smoking among the urban poor is of particular concern because low socioeconomic status puts individuals in this population at very high risk for the adverse effects of smoking.

- Access to health care in the urban poor is a critical public health issue, with large systematic barriers at play. The poor in general are additionally targeted by the tobacco companies by some of their biggest promotional offers.

- Clinical solutions for treatment of tobacco dependence are the same for the urban poor as in the general population, and include counseling and peer support, nicotine replacement therapy, and the use of pharmacotherapeutic agents such as bupropion and varenicline. However, patients also may be unable to afford prescribed medications or nicotine replacement therapy.

- Barriers to care for the urban poor must be considered when initiating a tobacco cessation plan. Culturally-sensitive self-help tobacco cessation literature and phone support may be effective strategies.

- Increases in tobacco taxation tend to decrease tobacco consumption in poorer populations, and tax monies raised can be aimed at media and other campaigns that promote tobacco cessation for this group.

Even though with taxation there is still disparity seen in the prevalence of smoking between different socioeconomic classes, taxation tends to narrow this gap. Increases in tobacco taxation may have a greater deleterious financial impact on the poor than on wealthier persons since they spend a higher percentage of their total income on cigarettes. However, the poor also carry a higher burden of disease that is a direct effect of tobacco use. The goal of cigarette taxation is to discourage all purchasers of tobacco products from continued use. Additionally, tax monies raised can be aimed at media and other campaigns that promote tobacco cessation, and these efforts can be particularly directed toward poorer populations. Policy makers have a duty to protect this particularly vulnerable population.

One New Zealand study calculated that a tax increase of 16% decreased the national rate of tobacco consumption over the following year by 10% [15]. Another study out of the United Kingdom found that as the price of cigarettes rose 342% over a 15 year period, from $3.39 to $11.60 ($US equivalents), the prevalence of smoking decreased somewhat more dramatically in poorer populations (36.5% to 28.4%) when compared to higher income groups (21.5% to 16.6%) [16]. Since increases in tobacco taxation are directly related to decreases in tobacco consumption, this appears to be the most effective of currently used strategies for global tobacco cessation.

REFERENCES

[1]   Mercado S, Havernann K, Sami M, Ueda H. Urban Poverty: An Urgent Public Health Issue. *Journal of Urban Health*. May 2007. 84(1):7-15.

[2]   Garau P, Sclar ED. Interim Report of the Millennium Development Goal Task Force 8 on Improving the Lives of Slum Dwellers. New York: United Nations; 2004.

[3]   Hyman DJ, Simons-Morton DG, Dunn JK, Ho K. Smoking, Smoking Cessation, and Understanding of the Role of Multiple Cardiac Risk Factors Among the Urban Poor. *Preventive Medicine*. 1996. 25: 653-659.

[4]   Diez-Roux AV, Nieto FJ, Muntaner C, Tyroler HA, Comstock GW, Shahar E, Cooper LS, Watson RL, Szklo M. Neighborhood Environments and Coronary Heart Disease: A Multilevel Analysis. *American Journal of Epidemiology*. 1997. 146(1): 48-63.

[5]   Lee, D. The Urban Poor's Economic Profile of Tobacco Use. *The American Journal of Drug and Alcohol Abuse*. 2008. 34: 626-633.

[6]   Kiefe CT, Hyman DJ. Do public clinic systems provide health care access for the urban poor? A cross-sectional survey. *Journal of Community Health.* 1996 Feb;21(1):61-70

[7]   Freeman HE, Corey CR. Insurance status and access to health services among poor persons. *Health Services Research.* 1993 Dec. 28(5):531-41.

[8]   Hyland A, Bauer JE, Li Q, Abrams SM, Higbee C, Peppone L, Cummings KM. Higher cigarette prices influence cigarette purchase patterns. *Tobacco Control.* 2005. 14:86-92

[9]   Federal Trade Commission Cigarette Report for 2004-2005. Acquired on May 30, 2009 at: http://www.ftc.gov/reports/tobacco/2007cigarette2004-2005.pdf.

[10] Feighery EC, Ribisl KM, Schleicher NC, Clark PI. Retailer participation in cigarette company incentive programs is related to increased levels of cigarette advertising and cheaper cigarette prices in stores. *Preventive Medicine.* June 2004. 38(6):876-884.

[11] Blumenthal DS. Barriers to the Provision of Smoking Cessation Services Reported by Clinicians in Underserved Communities. *Journal of the American Board of Family Medicine.* 2007. 20:272-279.

[12] Ahluwalia JS, McNagny SE, Clark WS. Smoking Cessation Among Inner-City African Americans Using the Nicotine Transdermal Patch. *Journal of General Internal Medicine.* 1998. 13(1):1-8.

[13] Resnicow K, Vaughan R, Futterman R, Weston RE, Royce J, Parms C, Hearn MD, Smith M, Freeman HP, Orlandi MA. A Self-Help Smoking Cessation Program for Inner-City African Americans: Results from the Harlem Health Connection Project. *Health Education and Behavior.* 1997. 24(2):201-17.

[14] Myung S-K, McDonell DD, Kazinets G, Seo HG, Moskowitz JM. Effects of Web- and Computer-Based Smoking Cessation Programs. Meta-analysis of Randomized Controlled Trials. *Archives of Internal Medicine.* May 25, 2009. 169(10):929-937.

[15] Wilson N, Thomson G. Tobacco tax as a health protecting policy: a brief review of the New Zealand evidence. *The New Zealand Medical Journal.* April 2005. 118(1213).

[16] Siahpush MS, Wakefield MA, Spittal MJ, Durkin SJ, Scollo MM. Taxation Reduces Social Disparities in Adult Smoking Prevalence. *American Journal of Preventive Medicine.* 2009. 36(4): 285-291.

Chapter 11

TOBACCO DEPENDENCE TREATMENT AND THE RURAL POOR

TOBACCO USE PATTERNS AND PUBLIC HEALTH IMPACT

Cigarette smoking is more prevalent among both adults and adolescents in rural regions than it is in suburban or urban communities. In rural areas, there is a 25% smoking prevalence rate, compared with 22% in urban communities and 21% in the general United States population [1]. Additionally, the overall decreased prevalence of smoking in the U.S. during the last 40 years has not seen as sharp of a decline in rural communities [2]. In some rural areas, the prevalence has actually seen increases by as much as two percentage points [3]. On average, the rural smoker also tends to consume more cigarettes per day [2].

The most rural counties in the American South have the highest regional rates of heart disease-related deaths for men and the second highest rates for women [4], [5]. Additionally, the smallest mortality declines for premature coronary heart disease among both white and African American persons are in these areas [5], [6]. Lung cancer rates are also higher among both white and African American males in certain rural areas in the South, such as Georgia, when compared to urban areas [7]. Poor survival from lung cancer in rural areas seems to be associated with low socioeconomic class and poor supply of health care providers [8].

POPULATION-SPECIFIC BARRIERS TO TREATMENT OF TOBACCO DEPENDENCE

Rural regions of the country face unique barriers to health care access related to geographic isolation. Patients (or families of patients) that are unable to take time off from work, that are housebound, that lack transportation access, who live in remote rural areas or regions with weather and terrain barriers, or who have no nearby providers may not be able to access the health care they need [9]. In other words, even if health care could be provided at low or no cost, that does not mean that a patient will be able to receive it. Rural communities are affected by greater distances from health care facilities, lower rates of health insurance coverage, inadequate access to specialty and mental health care, and limited options for smoking cessation programs and interventions [2].

A study involving rural communities in Kansas identified several individual barriers to smoking cessation, such as the belief that the damage from smoking was already done, that smoking is enjoyable and it helps with boredom and loneliness, and that tools that help with tobacco cessation may be of uncertain benefit [2]. Additional systematic barriers that were identified included inadequate finances to visit a physician, a paucity of local cessation programs, and poor knowledge about available products and services for quitting [2]. Other community-related and social factors also played a role. These included a lack of alternative activities to smoking, the absence of public smoking restrictions, and having friends and family who smoke [2]. In addition, patients from rural areas were less likely than those from urban settings to report that they received consistent advice and assistance on smoking cessation from their physicians [2].

CLINICAL SOLUTIONS

For low-income rural populations, telephone-based tobacco quit lines can be of significant benefit because these work around the need for traveling to physician visits and can be offered as a free service. The hours for quit lines can also be flexible so that participants can use the program despite work and childcare obligations. Telephone quit lines provide individualized assistance to patients and have been shown improve cessation rates [10].

Other clinical solutions for treating tobacco cessation in the rural poor include internet- and email-based counseling programs and telemedicine. These are all cost-effective solutions for bringing tobacco education and cessation counseling to geographical areas that have poor access to health care [2]. Nicotine replacement therapy is important for cessation in rural populations as it can be purchased over the counter and may be readily accessible. However the utility of this recommendation may be limited by its associated expense. Cost also limits the access of pharmacological interventions such as bupropion and varenicline, although these medications may be very helpful for patients in rural areas.

KEY POINTS

- Cigarette smoking is more prevalent in rural regions than in suburban or urban communities. The overall decreased prevalence of smoking in the U.S. over the last 40 years has not seen as sharp of a decline in rural communities, and some rural areas are actually seeing increased prevalence of tobacco use.

- The greatest barriers to assisting the rural poor with tobacco cessation appear to be related to decreased access to adequate care and a limited education about tobacco cessation programs/resources and their effectiveness.

- Patients in rural areas may be unable to access or afford prescribed medications or nicotine replacement therapy. Telephone counseling, internet and email based programs, and telemedicine are practical solutions to assist patients with tobacco cessation.

HEALTH POLICY RECOMMENDATIONS

The greatest barriers to assisting the rural poor with tobacco cessation appear to be related to decreased access to adequate care and a limited education about tobacco cessation programs and resources. Currently several programs exist to improve primary medical care to rural areas in the United States, such as the National Health Service Corps and the Indian Health Service. Providers are often incentivized to join these programs by being given significant reductions in their student loan debt. The Health Resources and Services Administration (HRSA) branch of the U.S. Department of Health and Human Services also provides a number of grants and training opportunities for rural health care, particularly through the Office of Rural Health Policy (ORHP). Improved access to motivated, well-trained providers will help to promote tobacco cessation programs and other critical health care initiatives in rural regions. Educational programs, offered to youth at early ages in the public school system, can also be used to help educate them about avoiding the initiation of smoking altogether. Drug programs that offer discounted or free medications would also be helpful in this population.

REFERENCES

[1]   U.S. Centers for Disease Control and Prevention (CDC), "Cigarette Smoking in Adults – -- United States 2006." *Morbidity and Mortality Weekly Report (MMWR)*. November 9, 2007. 56(44):1157-1161. Acquired on June 4, 2009 at: http://www.cdc.gov/mmwr/preview /mmwrhtml /mm5644a2.htm.

[2]   Hutcheson T, Greiner KA, Ellerbeck E. Understanding smoking cessation in rural communities. *The Journal of Rural Health*. 2008. 24(2):116-124.

[3]   Doescher MP, Jackson JE, Jerant A, Hart L. Prevalence and Trends in Smoking: A National Rural Study. *The Journal of Rural Health*. 2006. 22(2):112-118.

[4]   Eberhardt M, Ingram D, Makuc D, Pamuk ER, Freid VM, Harper SB, Schoenborn CA, Xia H. Urban and Rural Health Chartbook. *Health United States, 2001*. Hyattsville, MD: National Center for Health Statistics, 2001.

[5]   Zuniga M, Anderson D, Alexander K. (2003). Heart Disease and Stroke in Rural America. Rural Healthy People 2010: A companion document to Healthy People 2010. Volume 1. College Station, TX: The Texas A&M

University System Health Science Center, School of Rural Public Health, Southwest Rural Health Research Center. Retrieved May 25, 2009 from http://www.srph.tamhsc.edu/centers/rhp2010/06Volume1heart.htm

[6]   Barnett E, Halverson J. Disparities in premature coronary heart disease mortality by region and urbanicity among black and white adults ages 35-64, 1985-1995. *Public Health Reports.* 2000. 115(1):52-64.

[7]   Singh S, Bayakly AR, McNamara C, Redding K. Lung Cancer in Georgia, 1999-2002. Georgia Department of Human Resources, Division of Public Health, Chronic Disease, Injury, and Environmental Epidemiology Section. February, 2005. Publication number DPH06/006W.Retrieved May 25, 2009 from http://health.state.ga.us/pdfs/chronic/cancer/lungCancer99_02.pdf.

[8]   Shugarman LR, Sorbero MES, Tian H, Jain AK, Ashwood JS. An Exploration of Urban and Rural Differences in Lung Cancer Survival Among Medicare Beneficiaries. *American Journal of Public Health.* July 2008. 98(7):1280-1287.

[9]   Friedman E. Money isn't everything. Nonfinancial barriers to access. *JAMA.* May 18, 1994. 271(19):1535-8.

[10] Gollust S, Schroeder S, Warner K. Helping Smokers Quit: Understanding the Barriers to Utilization of Smoking Cessation Services. *The Milbank Quarterly.* 2008. 86(4):601-627.

Chapter 12

TOBACCO DEPENDENCE TREATMENT IN THE ILLITERATE

TOBACCO USE PATTERNS AND PUBLIC HEALTH IMPACT

There are an estimated 42 million U.S. adults who cannot read and an additional 50 million who are considered to be functionally illiterate, reading below the 5th grade level [1]. As one in four teenagers drop out of high school annually, and one in four of those who remain in school only reach the equivalent of an 8th grade education, it is estimated that the number of functionally illiterate Americans is growing by 2.25 million persons per year [1]. Literacy level has a significant effect on health care. In a study of patients at two public hospitals, a large number were deemed to have functional health illiteracy as they were unable to read and comprehend basic medical instructions – totalling 35% of all English-speaking and 61% of all Spanish-speaking patients [2]. In the patient groups examined, 41% of individuals were unable to understand directions for taking a prescription on an empty stomach, 26% could not understand when their next appointment was scheduled, 59% could not understand a standard informed consent document, 23% could not understand how to take a prescription four times per day, and 81% could not understand the rights and responsibilities of a Medicaid application. Data from this and other studies [3] suggest that the elderly are the highest at-risk group with regard to literacy status – up to 80% of both English- and Spanish-speaking patients are considered to read at a low literacy level.

Findings such as these suggest that literacy plays a major role in public health. The illiterate and non-English speaking subjects should generally not be excluded from research studies based on the fundamental principles of the Belmont Report. However, research inclusive of the illiterate may be limited by an inability to provide true informed consent, or in the fact that participants may avoid participation in survey-based research out of fear or embarrassment. There has not been much research specifically into the tobacco use patterns in the illiterate population, hence the public health impact of smoking in this population is not truly known. Even in the most recent data from the Centers for Disease Control [4], the prevalence rates of tobacco use were classified in many ways, but the closest category to illiteracy was education level (*see Figure 12.1*). In that data, smoking prevalence was found to be highest among adults who had earned a General Educational Development (GED) diploma (46.0%) or who had only 9 to 11 years of formal education (35.4%), and prevalence of tobacco use decreased as individuals' education levels increased. Since, as mentioned previously, up to one in four teenagers who remain in high school only reach the equivalent of an 8th grade education [1], and 18% of people with low literacy hold a high school diploma [3], education level and degree literacy do not perfectly correlate. In one study at a public hospital clinic, the reading levels of smokers and the readability of smoking cessation materials was examined [5]. In this study group, the participants' number of years completed in school was not a reliable predictor of their reading ability.

POPULATION-SPECIFIC BARRIERS TO TREATMENT OF TOBACCO DEPENDENCE

A significant amount of patient educational resources and media-based tobacco cessation campaigns are provided via printed educational materials. This approach will clearly have limited effect on the illiterate and functionally illiterate. Health care literature is generally written at the 10th grade level or above [6]. It has been found that up to 30-50% of the target audience for these materials is unable to read at this level, and therefore is unable to understand the message [6]. Additionally, misconceptions on the part of health care providers may play a role, including those that illiterate persons are likely to be poor, intellectually-impaired, immigrants, minorities, or that they will forthcoming about their inability to read [3]. In terms of absolute numbers, low literacy levels are actually more common in white, native-born Americans [3]. Health care providers must recognize the problems associated with care for persons with low literacy, and take pro-active steps to address tobacco cessation specifically in this population.

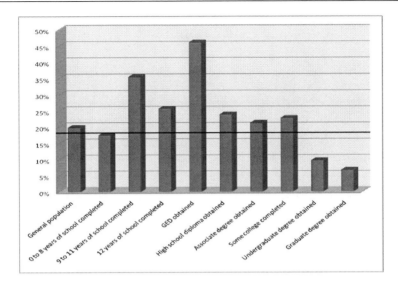

Figure 12.1. By 2006 data, the estimated percentage of adults (persons > 18 years of age) who are current smokers, as differentiated by education level. A horizontal bar represents the national current smoking rate for all races and all genders combined (19.8%). Source: U.S. Centers for Disease Control and Prevention (CDC), "Cigarette Smoking in Adults – -- United States 2006." Morbidity and Mortality Weekly Report (MMWR). 56(44):1157-1161, November 9, 2007, Acquired on June 4, 2009 at: http://www.cdc.gov/mmwr/preview/mmwrhtml/mm5644a2.htm.

CLINICAL SOLUTIONS

Clinical solutions for treating tobacco cessation in the low literacy and illiterate patient population include the use of group support, cognitive behavioral therapy, nicotine replacement therapy, and pharmacologic treatment such as bupropion and varenicline. These recommendations are based on those for the general population as there have been no studies on tobacco cessation that specifically target low-literacy persons. It is important for the physician to assess their patient's literacy status and tailor their recommendations for these patients to a lower reading level. This may include having educational handouts that are largely pictorial. Group and individual sessions for cognitive behavioral therapy could be successful in this population as they are discussion-based. Patients with low levels of literacy may also need individual demonstration of the proper use of nicotine replacement therapy agents and other medications, and not be left to rely on written instructional materials.

KEY POINTS

• Over 90 million Americans are considered illiterate or functionally illiterate. Literacy level has a significant effect on health care. Up to 30-50% of the target audience for tobacco cessation materials is unable to adequately read them or understand their message. Additionally, misconceptions on the part of health care providers about low literacy persons may play a role.

• Group support and cognitive behavioral therapy, nicotine replacement therapy, and pharmacologic treatment with bupropion and varenicline are all recommended for persons with low literacy levels.

• Educational handouts for this patient population should be largely pictorial. Group and individual sessions for cognitive behavioral therapy could be helpful in this population as they are discussion-based. Individual demonstration of the proper use of nicotine replacement therapy agents and other medications may be necessary.

• Health policy strategies for this population include educating health care providers to better identify persons with low literacy levels, and improving patient education styles and informative materials to better meet the needs of these individuals.

HEALTH POLICY RECOMMENDATIONS

There are a number of national campaigns to address literacy in general. It appears that initiatives to inform health care providers on how to identify and address the needs of persons with low literacy levels will be key to improved patient counseling and education, medication adherence/compliance and error reduction, means of obtaining informed consent, and perhaps even improved access to and utilization of payer sources such as Medicaid. Revision of forms and printed materials, including those present in medication packaging, must be done to consider the needs of low literacy persons. Experts in literacy, and specifically health care literacy, can be utilized to break down systematic barriers to care for this vulnerable patient population. All of these policy movements for health care in general can also be applied specifically to tobacco cessation campaigns.

REFERENCES

[1] Sweet RW. Illiteracy: An Incurable Disease or Education Malpractice? 1996. The National Right to Read Foundation. Retrieved May 27, 2009 from http://www.nrrf.org/essay_Illiteracy.html.

[2] Williams MV, Parker RM, Baker DW, Parikh NS, Pitkin K, Coates WC, Nurss JR. Inadequate Functional Health Literacy Among Patients at Two Public Hospitals. *JAMA*. 1995. 274(21): 1677-1682.

[3] Roter D, Rude R, Comings J. Patient Literacy: A Barrier to Quality of Care. *Journal of General Internal Medicine*. 1998 December. 13(12): 850-851.

[4] U.S. Centers for Disease Control and Prevention (CDC), "Cigarette Smoking in Adults – -- United States 2006." *Morbidity and Mortality Weekly Report (MMWR)*. November 9, 2007. 56(44):1157-1161. Acquired on June 4, 2009 at: http://www.cdc.gov/mmwr/preview /mmwrhtml /mm5644a2.htm.

[5] Meade C, Byrd J. Patient Literacy and the Readability of Smoking Education Literature. *American Journal of Public Health*. Feb 1989. 79(2):204-206.

[6] Plimpton S, Root J. Materials and Strategies That Work in Low Literacy Health Communication. *Public Health Reports*. Jan-Feb 1994. 109(1):86-92.

Chapter 13

TOBACCO DEPENDENCE TREATMENT IN THOSE WITH COMORBID MENTAL ILLNESS

TOBACCO USE PATTERNS AND PUBLIC HEALTH IMPACT

Persons carrying a psychiatric diagnosis have a very high prevalence of concurrent tobacco abuse, with reported smoking rates in this population ranging from 52%-90% [1]. Treatment for mental health disorders in the previous year is associated with an Adjusted Odds Ratio for daily smoking of 1.16, for alcohol abuse or dependence of 1.86, and for illicit drug abuse or dependence of 2.80 [2]. The tobacco, alcohol, and illicit drug use in this population places this group at tremendous risk for the adverse health effects of these substances. However, there have not been significant research data reported that specifically examined the public health impact of smoking in this population.

POPULATION-SPECIFIC BARRIERS TO TREATMENT OF TOBACCO DEPENDENCE

Systematic barriers often prevent persons with mental illness from accessing the health care they need in general. Since its creation in 1965, the Medicaid program has significantly expanded access to mental health care for low-income patients, and mental health care represents a significant proportion of the Medicaid budget [3]. Medicaid assists patients with both the cost of acute and chronic care needs, as well as that for prescription drugs. Despite the Medicaid program's successes, patients with mental disorders still make up a disproportionately large subset of the uninsured population [3]. Persons who are uninsured are more likely to have not received any outpatient mental health care services prior to a first hospitalization for psychotic illness [4], suggesting a missed opportunity for care. A critical "take-home" point to be made is that insurance coverage of patients with mental illness does not ensure that they will have access to care [5] as many other issues are also at play. Persons with chronic mental illness or confusion may find it difficult to navigate an increasingly complex health care and insurance system [5]. Additionally, the social stigma of having mental illness, in combination with issues such as fear of coercive treatment [6], mistrust of the health care system [7], and even a belief in supernatural causation for one's mental illness [7], have all been shown to drive patients away from obtaining the psychiatric care they need.

The demographically highest rates of persons seeking mental health treatment in the U.S. are seen among adults aged 26 to 49, in women more than in men, in American Indians/Alaska Natives or persons reporting more than one race, in divorced and separated persons, in persons with at least some college education, in the unemployed, in habitants of small metropolitan areas, in those with less than $20,000 family income, and in members of families who receive government assistance [2]. Hence, patients with tobacco dependence and underlying mental illness may face additional cultural and systematic barriers to successful smoking cessation.

Another hindrance to smoking cessation in persons with psychiatric illness is their understanding of the harms of tobacco use. In one study of inpatients at a psychiatric facility, only 68% of the patients interviewed believed that smoking was harmful to their health and quitting would be beneficial to their health [1]. This is in contrast to national data that show 93.4% of the smoking population believes that smoking is harmful to their health [8], [9]. One of the first steps to tobacco cessation is contemplation of quitting, and often the main reason for this is health concerns. If persons with mental illness do not fully understand the short- and long-term health effects of smoking, they may be less inclined to enter the contemplation phase of cessation. Mental illness is associated with fewer quit attempts and a lower cessation success rate than in the general population [10]. Additional factors include the perceptions of providers and mental health institutions that this population is unmotivated to quit smoking, lacks the cognitive function and necessary insight to quit smoking, and that tobacco cessation would take away one of the patient's only "pleasures" [1].

Persons with depression have a high prevalence of smoking and a low likelihood of quitting successfully [11]. And conversely, major depression is present in 6.6% of smokers and 2.9% of nonsmokers. Smokers carrying a diagnosis of depression only have a 14% success rate in smoking cessation attempts [11]. Nicotine may play a role in these findings as it may have the benefit of reducing negative affect [1] and increasing the release of dopamine in the brain [12]. Smoking may also complicate the treatment of depression, as it has been shown to decrease the blood levels of some antidepressants [1]. In addition, hepatic microsomal enzymes are activated by nicotine and tar, increasing the metabolism of neuroleptic medications and hence blunting the effect of these medications [12]. Therefore these medications need to be titrated to effect more closely in smokers. As tobacco actually improves some of the symptoms experienced by persons with psychiatric disorders, nicotine withdrawal can lead to exacerbation of some psychiatric disorders [10]. Smokers also have two to three times' higher risk of tardive dyskinesia with dopamine-blocking neuroleptic drugs, perhaps due to the higher doses that are required by smokers or to the increased dopaminergic activity induced by nicotine [13]. All of these factors need to be taken into account by health care providers that treat smokers with a psychiatric diagnosis.

CLINICAL SOLUTIONS

In patients with psychiatric illness, clinical recommendations for treating tobacco dependence include the use of cognitive behavioral therapy, nicotine replacement therapy, and bupropion. Nortriptyline has also been studied in patients with psychiatric illness who smoke – a small trial in 2004 showed that adding nortriptyline to nicotine replacement therapy and counseling resulted in a 50% reduction in smoking at one year [14]. In patients with major depression, integration of cognitive behavioral therapy with standard smoking cessation treatment has the greatest success [15]. Bupropion has also been studied in patients with depression and has been shown to improve smoking cessation rates [14]. In patients with schizophrenia, atypical antipsychotics in combination with nicotine replacement therapy or bupropion may be efficacious [15].

It is important to note that the use of any pharmacotherapeutic agent for tobacco cessation must be done with caution and vigilance in patients with underlying psychiatric illness. All patients on varenicline, including those with underlying mental illness, must be monitored for side effects such as agitation, depressed mood, atypical changes in behavior, or suicidal thoughts and behavior [16]. Patients with depression or other mental illnesses may have suicidal thoughts, and must be watched very closely for clinical worsening when taking antidepressant medications, including bupropion [17] and nortriptyline [18], especially early in their treatment or when their dose is adjusted.

KEY POINTS

• Persons carrying a psychiatric diagnosis have a high prevalence of concurrent tobacco abuse, with reported smoking rates in this population ranging from 52%-90%.

• Systematic barriers often prevent persons with mental illness from accessing the health care they need in general. Additional cultural barriers may play a role, and persons with psychiatric illness may have less insight into the harms of tobacco use. Better access to mental health care and psychiatric medications is essential to mental health policy in general. Greater incorporation of tobacco cessation into mental health visits, inpatient psychiatric treatment plans, and substance abuse programs is key.

• The chemicals in cigarettes affect brain neurochemistry and the metabolism of psychiatric drugs in a way that makes management of both the underlying mental illness and tobacco dependence more challenging.

• Clinical recommendations for treating tobacco dependence include cognitive behavioral therapy and nicotine replacement therapy. Nortriptyline may be another viable option. However, caution must be used with bupropion, varenicline, and nortriptyline in this population as worsening of psychiatric symptoms may occur.

HEALTH POLICY RECOMMENDATIONS

It used to be the case that patients in inpatient psychiatric facilities were allowed to smoke, and smoking breaks were actually used as a reward for good behavior [40]. Over the past several years there has been more research into smoking and mental illness. Studies have shown that bans on smoking for patients going through substance abuse and alcohol treatment programs actually increase the interest and success in quitting substance abuse and alcohol abuse [19], [20]. Over the past few years, as more hospitals have banned smoking for inpatients, so have mental health facilities. This is an important step to decreasing the acceptability of smoking by health care professionals. Smoking cessation in the inpatient setting can be beneficial because of the existing network of support (such as counseling), the availability of nicotine replacement and other medications, and the provision of a social environment that does not pressure an individual to restart smoking.

Tobacco dependence treatment is especially challenging in persons with mental illness. Even though the majority of persons with mental illness realize that smoking is detrimental to their health, there is generally less insight into this than in the general population. Additionally, mental illness is associated with fewer quit attempts and a lower cessation success rate than in the general population. Better access to mental health care and psychiatric medications is essential to mental health policy in general. Greater incorporation of tobacco cessation into mental health visits, inpatient psychiatric treatment plans, and substance abuse programs will likely have a significant impact on smoking prevalence rates.

REFERENCES

[1]   Carosella A, Ossip-Klein D, Owens C. Smoking Attitudes, Beliefs, and Readiness to change among Acute and Long Term Care inpatients with psychiatric diagnoses. *Addictive Behaviors*. 1999. 24(3):331-344.

[2]   Prevalence of Mental Health Treatment among Demographic and Socioeconomic Subgroups. Demographic and Socioeconomic Characteristics of Adults Receiving Mental Health Treatment. SAMHSA, Office of Applied Studies, National Household Survey on Drug Abuse, 2000 and 2001. U.S. Department of Health and Social Services, Office of

Applied Studies website. Acquired on February 15, 2009 at: http://www.oas.samhsa.gov/ mhtx/ch2.htm#2.3.1

[3] Frank RG. Goldman HH. Hogan M. Medicaid and mental health: be careful what you ask for. *Health Affairs*. 2003 Jan-Feb. 22(1):101-13.

[4] Rabinowitz J, Bromet EJ, Lavelle J, Severance KJ, Zariello SL, Rosen B. Relationship between type of insurance and care during the early course of psychosis. *American Journal of Psychiatry*. 1998 Oct. 155(10):1392-7.

[5] Friedman E. Money isn't everything. Nonfinancial barriers to access. *JAMA*. May 18, 1994. 271(19):1535-8.

[6] Hahm HC, Segal SP. Failure to seek health care among the mentally ill. *American Journal of Orthopsychiatry*. 2005 Jan. 75(1):54-62.

[7] Chadda RK, Agarwal V, Singh MC, Raheja D. Help seeking behaviour of psychiatric patients before seeking care at a mental hospital. *International Journal of Social Psychiatry*. 2001. 47(4):71-8.

[8] Fiore MC, Bailey WC, Cohen SF. 2000. Treating Tobacco Use and Dependence: A Clinical Practice Guideline. Rockville, MD. U.S. Department of Health and Human Services.

[9] US Department of Health and Human Services. The health consequences of smoking: nicotine addiction. A report of the Surgeon General. Atlanta (GA): US Department of Health and Human Services. Public Health Service, Centers for Disease Control, Center for Chronic Disease Prevention and Health Promotion, Office of Smoking and Health. DHHS Publication No. (PHS) (CDC) 88-8406. 1988.

[10] Fagerstrom K, Aubin HJ. Management of smoking cessation in patients with psychiatric disorders. *Current Medical Research and Opinion*. 2009 Feb. 25 (2): 511-8.

[11] Glassman, AH. Cigarette Smoking: Implications for Psychiatric Illness. *American Journal of Psychiatry*. April 1993. 150(4): 546-553.

[12] Salokangas RK, Saarijarvi S, Taimien T, Lehto H, Niemi H, Alola V, Syvalahti E. Effect of Smoking on Neuroleptics in Schizophrenia. *Schizophrenia Research*. 1997. 23: 55-60.

[13] Binder,RL, Kazamatsuri H, Nishimura T, McNiel D. Smoking and Tardive Dyskinesia. *Biological Psychiatry*. 1987. 22(10): 1280-1282.

[14] Hall SM, Tsoh JY, Prochaska JJ, Eisendrath S, Rossi JS, Redding CA, Rosen AB, Meisner M, Humgleet GL, Gorecki JA. Treatment for Cigarette Smoking Among Depressed Mental Health Outpatients: A Randomized Clinical Trial. *American Journal of Public Health*. 2006. 96(10):1808-14.

[15] Kisely S, Campbell LA. Use of Smoking Cessation Therapies in Individuals with Psychiatric Illness : An Update for Prescribers. *CNS Drugs*. 2008. 22(4):263-73.

[16] Prescribing Information: CHANTIX® (varenicline) Tablets. Dosage and Administration. Retrieved May 17, 2009 from https://www.pfizerpro.com /sites/pfp/pages/product_info/Chantix_pi_dosage_and_adminiadminist.aspx Bupropion hydrochloride drug information. Retrieved May 17, 2009 from http://www.fda.gov/cder/drug/infopage/bupropion/default.htm.

[17] Nortriptyline. Drugs.com Drug Information Online. Acquired June 2, 2009 at: http://www.drugs.com/pro/nortriptyline.html.

[18] Joseph AM, Nichol KL, Willenbring ML, Korn JE. Beneficial effects of treatment of nicotine dependence during an inpatient substance abuse treatment program. *JAMA*. 1990. 263:3043-3046.

[19] Miller WR, Hedrick KE, Taylor CA. Addictive Behaviors and Life Problems Before and After Behavioral Treatment of Problem Drinkers. *Addictive Behaviors*. 1983. 8: 403-412.

Chapter 14

TOBACCO DEPENDENCE TREATMENT IN THE UNDER- AND UNINSURED

TOBACCO USE PATTERNS AND PUBLIC HEALTH IMPACT

As of January 2010, and hence before any formal plan for a U.S. government-sponsored national health insurance system has been implemented, there is an estimated 15.3% rate of uninsured persons in the United States – totaling 45.7 million people without insurance – and this number appears to be growing [1]. Approximately two-thirds of the uninsured are low-income individuals and families [2]. Uninsured status is highest in African Americans, Hispanics, persons aged 18 to 29, those with incomes of less than $25000 annually, the self-employed, and the unemployed [3]. Studies suggest that the prevalence of tobacco abuse is higher amongst the under- and uninsured (estimated at 39%) than in the general population (estimated at 21-23%) [4], [5].

Given the wide range of serious adverse health effects from smoking, and the limited access to health care amongst the under- and uninsured, the public health impact of tobacco use in this population is significant. Although there are no perfect estimates of the true financial impact of all tobacco-related health problems, almost half of all such costs are thought to be covered by federal programs (such as Medicare and Medicaid), and approximately $38 billion in federal tax dollars are spent yearly on this alone – the equivalent of $320 in annual federal taxes per household [6]. This does not take into consideration the cost of health care for persons without a payer source at all. Beyond cost, low-income smokers suffer more health complications from tobacco because of greater tobacco use. Additionally, persons working in "blue collar" jobs are also more likely to be exposed to second-hand smoke [6]. Limited access to health care due to under- and uninsured status also means that persons in this group are more likely to be diagnosed at advanced stages of tobacco-related illness and will therefore ultimately need greater amounts of health care services [7]. Reports also suggest that this population tends overall to receive poor quality health services, and that many ultimately go without treatment at all [8].

POPULATION SPECIFIC BARRIERS TO TREATMENT

Barriers to treatment of tobacco abuse in the under- and uninsured are similar to those of the rural and urban poor, which have been previously reviewed. Overall, there is decreased access to health care services as a result of an inability to pay for those services, and an inability to afford the recommended treatments to assist with cessation. In addition, although the under- and uninsured population has a higher prevalence of tobacco use, some studies suggest that these patients, even when able to access outpatient health care, tend to receive less counseling on tobacco cessation [4]. It is felt that this inequity is due in part to decreased access to cessation interventions, and also due to the lesser quality of care that underserved patients often receive.

CLINICAL SOLUTIONS

Clinical solutions to improving the cessation rate of the under- and uninsured who smoke include increasing the access to tobacco cessation counseling on telephone quit lines and also through community outreach and support. There also needs to be increased access to primary care and drug assistance programs so that these persons can receive tobacco cessation counseling, nicotine replacement, and opportunities to benefit from pharmacotherapeutics such as bupropion and varenicline. There have been no specific studies targeting tobacco cessation treatment in people who are under- and uninsured, but more research needs to be done to improve the care provided to this population.

KEY POINTS

• There are around 45.7 million people in the U.S. without insurance and this number is growing. The prevalence of tobacco abuse is higher amongst the under- and uninsured (estimated at 39%) than in the general population (estimated at 23%).

• This group has decreased access to health care services and an inability to afford recommended treatments. Also, some data suggests that underserved patients often receive lower quality health services.

• Clinical recommendations for treating tobacco dependence are similar to those for the general population and include cognitive behavioral therapy, nicotine replacement therapy, bupropion, and varenicline. Tobacco cessation counseling on telephone quit lines and community outreach and support are options for those with particularly limited resources.

• Assisting those who qualify for government-funded health insurance will improve access to primary care, preventive services, and tobacco cessation interventions.

HEALTH POLICY RECOMMENDATIONS

A study performed by the Kaiser Commission found that close to 25% of the approximately 46.1 million (non-elderly) Americans who are uninsured, or around 11.5 million persons in total, actually qualified for government funded health insurance but were simply not enrolled [2],[9]. Barriers to enrolling these persons in health care programs must be identified and broken down – and this should be a major public health priority. Costs put forward to increase enrollment in health insurance programs would likely result in significant cost savings in return, particularly by improving access to primary care and preventive services. Policy changes are key to improving the access to care for under- and uninsured patients.

As discussed in previous sections, increased tobacco taxation may in the long-term be of particular benefit to persons in lower socioeconomic groups, as taxation tends to result in decreased tobacco consumption [10]. In January of 2008, the state of Indiana raised the tax on cigarettes and used that money to fund preventative services such as tobacco cessation programs, incentives for small business to offer health insurance to employees, and a plan to allow employers and employees to purchase health insurance on a pre-tax basis [11]. This is a good example of how an increase of tax on cigarettes can both discourage tobacco use and direct money to programs that increase access to health coverage and hence tobacco cessation programs.

REFERENCES

[1]   U.S. Census Bureau. Income, Poverty, and Health Insurance Coverage in the United States: 2007. Issued August 2008. Retrieved April 7, 2009 from: http://www.census.gov/prod/2008pubs/p60-235.pdf.

[2]   Urban Institute and Kaiser Commission on Medicaid and the Uninsured, analysis of March 2002 Current Population Survey. 2002. Retrieved May 17, 2009 from http://www.kff.org/uninsured/loader. cfm?url=/commonspot /security/getfile.cfmandPageID=14185.

[3]   Nelson DE, Bolen J, Wells HE, Smith SM, Bland S. State Trends in Uninsurance Among Individuals Aged 18-64 Years: United States, 1992-2001. *American Journal of Public Health*. 2004. 94(11): 1992-97.

[4]   Parnes B, Main D, Holcomb S, Pace W. Tobacco Cessation Counseling Among Underserved Patients: A Report from CaReNet. *The Journal of Family Practice*. 2002. 51(1): 65-69.

[5] U.S. Centers for Disease Control and Prevention (CDC). "Self-assessed Health Status and Selected Behavioral Risk Factors Among Persons With and Without Health-care Coverage- United States, 1994-1995. Morbidity and Mortality Weekly Report. 1998. 47(9): 176-180. Retrieved June 2, 2009 from http://www.cdc.gov/mmwr/preview/mmwrhtml/00051507.htm.

[6] National Center for Tobacco-Free Kids. Campaign for Tobacco-Free Kids. Factsheets. Acquired on April 7, 2009 at: http://www.tobaccofreekids.org/research/factsheets/.

[7] Adler, NE, Boyce WT, Chesney MA, Folkman S, Syme SL. Socioeconomic inequalities in health: No easy solution. *JAMA*. 1993. 269:3140-5.

[8] Fiscella K, Franks P, Gold MR, Clancy CM. Inequality in quality: Addressing socio-economic, racial, and ethnic disparities in health care. *JAMA*. May 17, 2000. 283(19):2579-2584.

[9] Dubay L, Holahan J, Cook A. The Uninsured And The Affordability Of Health Insurance Coverage. *Health Affairs*. 2007. 26: w22-w30.

[10] Myung S-K, McDonell DD, Kazinets G, Seo HG, Moskowitz JM. Effects of Web- and Computer-Based Smoking Cessation Programs. Meta-analysis of Randomized Controlled Trials. *Archives of Internal Medicine*. May 25, 2009. 169(10):929-937.

[11] "Healthy Indiana Plan" to Go Live in January. No author listed. *Healthcare Financial Management*. 2007. 61(10):13-14.

Chapter 15

TOBACCO DEPENDENCE TREATMENT AND SYSTEMATIC BARRIERS: CONCLUSIONS

The burden of tobacco-related diseases is inequitably divided, with a disproportionate share falling upon those with inadequate resources and poor access to quality health care. Limitations to health care access occur for various reasons – comorbid illness, financial hardship, insurance status, geographic barriers, resource availability, sociocultural factors, and decreased ability to navigate through an increasingly complex health care system. And for unclear reasons, the degree of tobacco counseling and cessation assistance offered to patients of limited means tends to be less than that for other patients. While access to affordable tobacco products exists, fair access to the treatment of tobacco dependence does not.

To successfully make an impact on the public health burden of tobacco in underserved patient populations, far greater outreach must be done. Tobacco taxation is a proven method to decrease smoking prevalence rates. Increasing the availability of medications and other cessation services to those of limited means or access can be done with the collected tax revenues. Banning smoking in the workplace, schools, and other public areas will likely have a significant impact. Expanding free services which have been shown to be effective, such as telephone- and internet-based counseling, can be done for those with cost, geographic, language, literacy, or time barriers. And incentivizing health care providers to train and work in programs, such as the National Health Service Corps, will improve the quality of health care for people living in isolated regions. Through concerted efforts, large strides can be made in combating this preventable disease that results in substantial mortality, disability, and spent resources.

INDEX